I STILL
DISAGREE

2ND EDITION

DR. PATRICK FLYNN, D.C.
Chiropractor

With contributing authors
Christy Flynn and Nicole Saleske FNP-BC, APNP

Published by Dr. Patrick Flynn, Green Bay, Wisconsin
Sale date and price under consideration

For more information, please contact:
The Wellness Way
2525 W. Mason Street
Green Bay, WI 54303
Visit us online at www.thewellnessway.com
To contact Dr. Patrick Flynn for speaking engagements visit
www.drpatrickflynn.com

ISBN: 979-8-88-344957-3

ACKNOWLEDGEMENTS

A project like this doesn't just happen. It takes a team of dedicated people to read, reread, edit, give feedback and reread again. I'd like to thank my team who rallied to make this project a success:

Jen Beh, Miranda Biebel, Jeremy Cookson, Brent Deterding, Dana Dilling, Deanna Ducat, Sara Frisque, Lauryn Gindl, Joi Gratny, Diana Guy, Stefanie Hushour, Erin Krueger, Travis Kunze, Dr. Zach Papendieck, Heidi Robeson, Nicole Saleske, Nicole Seidel, Betsy Schroeder, Luke Sonnleitner, Uriah Stutzman, Hayley Takis, Nathaniel Takis, Dennette Tallis, Erin Walton, Shelley Wank, Sarah Welsh, and my beautiful bride, Christy Flynn – I choose you.

I am very proud of my profession and study of chiropractic. The principles and philosophies I learned are the foundation of all I have done. Anytime I look at studies, data, and research, my training gives me insights to see things differently. I've heard many times, "You aren't a real doctor, you're just a chiropractor." I chuckle, shake my head, then go and continue to guide others as they change their lives with the health restoring principles based on simply physiology and chiropractic philosophy. I'm not just a chiropractor. I am a proud chiropractor.

With that in mind,

The material contained in this book is for informational purposes only and not to be used as medical or healthcare advice or guarantee of outcomes. Information has been gathered and shared from true stories, clinical examples, and reputable sources; however, Dr. Patrick Flynn, The Wellness Way, LLC, and entities connected with either are not responsible for errors or omissions. No individual, including those seeing a Wellness Way doctor, provider, or Health Restoration Coach should use the information, resources, or tools herein to self-diagnose or self-treat any health-related concerns. Information and statements made in this work are not intended to diagnose, treat, cure, or prevent any disease. For questions regarding your personal health concerns and conditions, please consult your doctor.

TABLE OF CONTENTS

PART 1

WHY I DISAGREE...
THE STORIES BEFORE
THE STORY.

CHAPTER 1

WHY DO I DISAGREE?

WHY DO I DISAGREE?

You've picked up this book and either know exactly what you are about to read or are about to be hit with a different perspective. Let me explain. I've been going against the grain for over 30 years. Actually, if you ask my mom, she'd say it's longer than that, more like all my life. Just for simplicity's sake, let's keep it to how healthcare, or better yet, how symptom and illness management-based care, are handled in "modern, developed countries." Or any countries in which those countries have an influence.

We've all had those moments. Maybe it hits you in the shower, or maybe it runs through your mind while you're driving. It definitely hits you when your opinionated cousin won't stop talking at the family reunion! It's the thought that something is a bit off; it doesn't resonate. Maybe you can't even put your finger on it, but you know something isn't right. You know you disagree with what's happening.

Since 2020, many people have had a clearer vision as to what has been happening, and what doesn't seem right, and they are daring to disagree. Let's start how I like to start most discussions in which we need to find common ground and understanding. If you were to join my team for any of the trainings I do or attend any seminar I speak at, you'd see me start by laying out some definitions. Let's start there.

disagree [dis-uh-gree]

verb (used without object) To not have the same opinion or idea

Synonyms: To differ, dissent, object, argue

It frustrates people when you simply say, "I disagree." Want to really get them emotional? Say it calmly. It'll drive them nuts.

Just be ready to defend what you actually believe. Try doing it logically. Whoa, that is enough to send them into orbit! Have you ever felt like the black sheep either in your family, workplace, or simply in society these days? Today, when that happens, it's not uncommon to be silenced, ridiculed, or screamed at. Some of us even have a government agency show up at our house...but that's another story.

Throughout history, it wasn't uncommon for people to disagree. In fact, some of the best institutions of education were set up to not just teach their students what to think, but how to think. Those institutions developed in their students the ability to defend their positions articulately while debating others with differing opinions. How far we've come: Or rather, how far we've fallen.

From 2020-2023, the COVID fiasco revealed just how much disagreeing with the mainstream and government was not allowed. Now, I'm not saying COVID wasn't a real infection or that it wasn't dangerous for people. It absolutely was and still is. But let's be clear; they weren't telling us the whole story. It wasn't dangerous for every single person to the degree of severity in the ways they made it seem, and their "precautions" were not at all based on current science methodologies.

Do you really let the government make your family's healthcare decisions?

What really woke people up, though, was when it became blatantly obvious that the government and pharmaceutical companies thought they should have more control of the healthcare decisions for your family -- not just in annual or well-child checkups. Here is where I disagree and have been sharing thoughts with others that they need to also stand up. Seriously? Do you really let the government make your family's healthcare decisions? Apparently, there is still a part of the population that thinks this is acceptable.

For anyone who dared to disagree or not continue the party line set out by various governments around the world--including unelected health "officials," "experts," and other random philanthropists turned health gurus and food experts--cancellation was a real thing. Social media was taken down and censored, real experts were ridiculed and discredited as dangerous, and laws were bent, broken, and straight out ignored to push forward one agenda. Their message was loud and clear: We're right, and if you question us, you question science. They are the science.

Some stood up and said, "I disagree!" I had been disagreeing for so long I simply jumped in and said, "I still disagree!" People from all walks of life, on both sides of the aisle, with ranging income and education levels, and from all over the world dared to disagree. For some people, it was the first time they'd likely agreed with each other. For others, it became a hard dividing line between family members and lifelong friends.

Some people realized what was going on right away and started speaking out. For others, it took a little while, and as their freedoms were trampled and stolen, they began to join the dissension. For another group, it took the realization that what they were seeing in the hospitals they were working in, attempting to save lives, wasn't the same as what they heard from their administrators, the media, and so many of the "experts" we mentioned earlier. For them, they either stood their ground and lost it all, others lost their hospital privileges, practices, and even their licenses, or choosing to become part of the silent majority.

Do you know what's frustrating to me? A silent majority! Why, if you are the majority, or even if you aren't the majority but you have something good to stand up for, would you

Do you know what's frustrating to me? A silent majority!

ever be silent?! Lives and livelihoods were on the line! Because not enough people stood up, vaccines have now been approved,

1 / WHY DO I DISAGREE?

although proven dangerous and not at all effective. Businesses have gone bankrupt, lives were lost, families devastated, and the mental health crisis has soared to new levels.

I get it; many people were scared. And, when you're scared, you tend to do exactly what you're told. And that's what they were counting on: They used fear against the citizens of the world. For too many, it was too much to bear. But do you know what overcomes fear? Truth and knowledge. Oh, I know today there is a whole discussion around "truth." We'll save that for another book. When you are educated and informed, you're better able to stand up to tyranny. I'll give you a hint: If the education and information are free and easily accessible, I'd question it. Better yet, ignore it. Especially if you see it is sponsored by a drug company!

But, thanks to those who dared to stand in disagreement, mandates have been cancelled, workers have been rehired, lies exposed, and even deeper corruption is being brought to light. People are standing up to the government and companies who would benefit and want to make the healthcare choices for your family.

This is all a great start, but was it too little too late? Or the rumblings of a true revolution of thinking? What happens when they come for our freedoms again? Will the people who talk big about not letting this happen again actually follow through with what they say? Or will they once again back down from the fight to keep our freedoms? We need warriors to start preparing for battle now, because the battle never ended...it's just begun.

Think about all that you've been told, all the "experts" you've trusted.

I know, I know, COVID fatigue is a real thing. Let's change the subject. But I want you to look through a new lens as you read the rest of the book. Think about all that you've been told, all the "experts" you've trusted, and try to see how the

12

system that has been exposed has been in place for far longer than you may have realized. In fact, it's likely touched you and your loved ones in some devastating ways.

PEELING BACK THE LAYERS

We all know a couple who have been so desperate for a baby that they've spent tens of thousands of dollars on treatments. For too many, there is still no child. Maybe the couple is you and your spouse. The money invested is overwhelming, but the heartache is even more so. Let me ask you a question, though: Why is this so common?

We all have stories. Remember a time when you looked into a loved one's eyes only to hear that the doctors said surgery is the only answer? Or another prescription was going to be written to see if it might help? Or even how they were told that despite the obvious symptoms, there was nothing wrong with them? Remember how you felt? In spite of everything, did a voice in your head whisper "no"? That inkling of disagreement was there!

Every day the news stations are flooded with reports of how people are sicker than ever. How can we have the best

How many prescriptions does a person need to be *healthy*?

medical technologies and research, but people are still on an average of four prescriptions a day, NOT including the over-the-counter medications they take? How many prescriptions does a person need to be *healthy*?

Here's one more question for you: When is enough, enough? Would you agree that this is the best we have to offer ourselves, or would you disagree?

THE HISTORY OF MODERN MEDICINE

Anyone who knows me knows I'm a total history buff. Seriously, I learn and study so much history so that I can better understand people and how we've gotten to where we are today. If you thought COVID ticked you off, wait till you hear the history of modern medicine.

Have you ever heard of John D. Rockefeller? Yes, the oil tycoon. That's how he became the richest man in the world. The Rockefeller Foundation is the philanthropic organization developed by America's first billionaire. So, what does he have to do with modern medicine? Keep reading.

In the early 1900s, chemicals derived from oil were becoming so popular that even the waste products became nearly as profitable as the oil itself! At about this same time, scientists were gaining an understanding of vitamins and other nutrients. They thought maybe they could use the same manufacturing process that was developing everything from plastics to kerosene to create pharmaceutical drugs.[1] After all, natural substances like vitamins, nutrients, and minerals can't be patented under U.S. law, but drugs could be.

So, what does Rockefeller have to do with pharmaceuticals? He already owned the oil industry.[2] So he set his sights on influencing medicine around the world as well.[3,4]

1 Hess, Jeremy, Daniel Bednarz, Jaeyong Bae, and Jessica Pierce. "Petroleum and Health Care: Evaluating and Managing Health Care's Vulnerability to Petroleum Supply Shifts." American journal of public health, September 2011. https://www.ncbi.nlm.nih.gov/pmc/articles/PMC3154246/.

2 "Standard Oil," Encyclopædia Britannica, February 23, 2024, https://www.britannica.com/topic/Standard-Oil.

3 RF annual Report - 1939. Accessed February 27, 2024. https://www.rockefellerfoundation.org/wp-content/uploads/Annual-Report-1939-1.pdf.

4 "Annual Report 1915." Rockefeller Foundation, 2003. https://www.rockefellerfoundation.org/wp-content/uploads/RF-Annual-Report-1915-1.pdf.

5 Frohlich, Edward D. "Leadership in American Medicine as I See It: A Background in the Beginning." Ochsner journal, 2012. https://www.ncbi.nlm.nih.gov/pmc/articles/PMC3527854/.

In 1909, nearly half the schools that were teaching doctors were focusing on natural, herbal treatments passed down through the ages and from European and Native Americans who also shared their ancestral knowledge. In fact, many conditions that had been considered diseases were being recognized as deficiencies of key nutrients. That's right: They could be treated with unpatentable vitamins and readily available support from nutritional foods and herbs.

What to do? You read it earlier in this chapter: Discredit, demonize, ridicule, and punish those who used absolutely any method or message contrary to the agenda. When you are backed by rich men, that's not hard to do. Especially without modern-day information channels and platforms.

Let's look at another key player in the story: Andrew Carnegie. The great steel magnate and founder of The Carnegie Foundation was well respected, and his opinions carried much weight, likely due to its hefty donations--another tactic we see today. Both had an idea as to how healthcare should be handled. Conspiracy? Absolutely, but not in the way you may think.

I want to take you down a little rabbit trail, so follow me here for a moment. Let's look at the meaning of some keywords here. According to Oxford's Dictionary:

conspiracy [kuhn-spir-uh-see]
noun A secret plan by a group to do something unlawful or harmful.
Synonyms: plotting, collusion, intrigue, collaboration, covert schemes

Side note: Study the history of "conspiracy theory" before jumping to conclusions or allowing someone to try to degrade you with that label. The government playing with words to manipulate public opinion isn't new.

The Carnegie Foundation, at the request of the American Medical Association (AMA) and in agreement with

Rockefeller's views, launched an audit of the medical schools in the U.S. [5] Now, sure, there were some subpar schools teaching some questionable practices. But that wasn't their focus. They had a mission to take out the competition, remember? That's where Abraham Flexner comes into the picture. For the record, Abraham's brother, Simon Flexner was the first director for the Rockefeller Institute for Medical Research.[6] Coincidence?

Now, like some people who have somehow become "experts" today, again, think uneducated (in health or medicine, at least) philanthropists and government employees, elected or not, Flexner, Carnegie, and Rockefeller had no medical training.[7] Instead, Abraham Flexner was an educator with a bias toward the type of study he'd experienced while in Europe, namely what was common in Germany at the time. This bias would certainly impact his findings.[8] With no medical training! No problem! The Carnegie Foundation (also no medical training) assisted him in how he should evaluate these schools. How convenient.

Flexner visited every one of the 155 schools educating doctors across the United States. His analysis, the Flexner report, was published in 1910.[9] Medicine and healthcare would never be the same. In his report, Flexner criticized a majority of the schools he reviewed and called for higher standards. He also recommended closing 120 of them. What do you suppose those "standards" he recommended might have been?

Medicine and healthcare would never be the same.

Or maybe ask yourself, who would have profited the most from those standards?

Of course, Flexner did suggest adding more hands-on clinical work and research, which are great things, for sure! And if that's where it ended, I would agree that it was a great report. But remember who paid for the "study"? Using the same tricks we see today to help push legislation, large campaign donations and lobbyists, it's easy for rich men to have their agendas seem acceptable to politicians who don't understand healthcare. Seems that Washington was able to be bought, even back then.

What did those large donations buy them? How about the American Medical Association (AMA) in charge of overseeing medical education? That is certainly a powerful move. It all sounds official and respectable until you follow the money once again. Soon, allopathic medicine was the only acceptable form of medicine in the U.S. What is allopathic medicine? Columbia University defines it this way:

> *Allopathic medicine refers to a system in which medical doctors and other healthcare professionals (such as nurses, pharmacists, and therapists) treat symptoms and diseases using drugs, radiation, or surgery. Also called biomedicine, conventional medicine, mainstream medicine, orthodox medicine, and Western medicine.*

The majority of what today would be called schools of complementary and alternative medicines (CAM) (think homeopathy, chiropractic, osteopathy, and naturopaths) were shut down. Do you know which other area of healthcare was affected? Psychiatry. I wonder how much of the mental health crisis today could have been avoided. Flexner went on to write additional reports for the Carnegie and Rockefeller foundations. He went on to work for the General Education Board of the Rockefeller Foundation in 1912.[10]

6 "Flexner, Simon." Digital Commons @ RU. Accessed February 27, 2024. https://
    digitalcommons.rockefeller.edu/faculty-members/28/.

7 Anne-Emanuelle Birn, Philanthrocapitalism, past and present: The Rockefeller Foundation,
    the Gates Foundation, and the setting(s) of the international/ global health
    agenda. Hypothesis 2014, 12(1): e8, doi:10.5779/hypothesis. v12i1.229.

8 Duffy, Thomas P. "The Flexner Report--100 Years Later." The Yale journal of biology and
    medicine, September 2011. https://www.ncbi.nlm.nih.gov/pmc/
    articles/PMC3178858/.

9 Medical education in the United States and Canada. Accessed February 28, 2024. http://
    archive.carnegiefoundation.org/publications/pdfs/elibrary/Carnegie_Flexner_
    Report.pdf.

10 "Abraham Flexner: Work." Institute for Advanced Study, October 13, 2020. https://www.
    ias.edu/flexner-work.

So, let's recap: Identify a profitable market, purchase "studies" to prove the "science" you need to portray, and then silence the critics, dissenters, and disagreers by villainizing them and making them look like fools. Oooh, I hope this causes you to look at "studies" a bit differently! Follow the money, not the headlines.

For good measure, Rockefeller and Carnegie funded and donated large sums to schools committed to teaching allopathic methods. Schools that taught more traditional methods simply couldn't compete against the finances of the Carnegie Foundation and the weight of the Rockefeller name. In the end, following the Flexner report and the Rockefeller/Carnegie conspiracy, (remember our definition!) over half of the schools training doctors in the U.S. were closed.

Do you know the best way for businesses to stay profitable? Make sure there is always a demand for the products that line their pockets. How do you do that? Play on people's emotions. What is more emotional than fear of sickness or even death? Especially if it is your child, parent, spouse, or even yourself who is sick. What would you pay? Whatever it takes. They're counting on it.

What is more emotional than fear of sickness or even death?

But what if you could invest in health instead of sickness? That's an investment that pays dividends for as long as you live! And it's way less costly in many, many ways.

Have you woken up? Has your mind been blown? How about one last angle to glance at: Guess who founded the American Cancer Society in 1913? Actually, who is still funding large health initiatives today?[11] None other than the Rockefeller

11 "Our History." The Rockefeller Foundation, February 22, 2024. https://www. rockefellerfoundation.org/about-us/our-history/.
12 "Since Insurance's Humble Start in Dallas, Hospital Inflation Has Always Posed Challenge." Dallas News, August 26, 2019. https://www.dallasnews. com/business/2015/03/06/since-insurance-s-humble-start-in-dallas-hospital-inflation-has-always-posed-challenge/.

family. I wonder if donations would stop if there was a cure. Likely. What would happen if society knew that many cancers are lifestyle-driven and preventable? That free money would stop pouring in; I'm sure of it. But more on that in a later chapter.

Consider just how new "modern medicine" really is compared to other forms of healthcare. Compared to human history, modern medicine is truly in its infancy, or maybe the gangly teen years. But, make no mistake, it's a huge market full of expenses and profits. Knowing which side you are on is crucial.

THE ONLY THING COVERED BY INSURANCE IS THE INDUSTRY!

Remember the advice I shared earlier? When information and education are free and readily available, it may be better to run away from it. Let's apply that thought to healthcare. Universal healthcare has been a political debate for decades. Ask yourself why.

Shall we discuss the insurance industry, how they determine what is covered, and what isn't? Hospitals were designed for the poor and disabled. If you were wealthy, you'd get care at home. Hospitals are costly to run and maintain. Unfortunately, their expenses were naturally high and not really dependent upon how many patients they served. In Dallas, Texas, 1500 teachers paid fifty cents per month in 1929 to "insure" 14-21 days of care at Baylor University Hospital for any one of the contributors who needed it. Remember, most schoolteachers were single women at this time, and their incomes were roughly $2,000 per year. That $.50 a month could mean a lot if they didn't have local family to care for them while they were ill. This cash flow stabilized the income for the hospital.[12] However, only care provided in the hospital was covered. And the hospital was paid whether services were used or not. The fee-for-service plan (which led to more services and the ability to collect more fees) that evolved created concerns for insurance companies who began instituting barriers to coverage from pre-existing conditions to auditing bills.[12] Because many of the early plans that soon followed were dedicated to specific hospitals, consumers didn't have to shop around. They basically had two options. Take it or leave it. From there, the spiral began. But I'm not here to educate you on the ins and outs of insurance. Want to know why?

I'd rather make a choice in care. True freedom is when you have the freedom to choose how you care for your health, and unfortunately, the promise of saving money with insurance does not equate to saving lives. In fact, insurance companies often limit the services doctors who are trained in restoring health over symptom management are able to provide…if they cover them at all! Remember, there is no profit in health, only in managing sickness.

I know that was a lot to take in. But you have to know the history of the industry to understand how we got to where we are today. It's not just COVID that was used to play with our emotions and, worse yet, our health, healthcare choices, and personal freedoms. Yes, the government and the drug companies are conspiring on this. This has been going on for generations. Here's one more example for you.

1986 ACT

I love technology and innovation. In my clinics and headquarters, everyone knows I can't stand crappy tools. I want my team to have the best of the best so that we can produce the best of the best.

Think of a conversation you may have had with your grandparents and what health and medicine looked like when they were younger. Now, I know what you are thinking, Doc, there have been so many advances. I'm so happy I live today! Now think about that same conversation with your grandparents and how they always seem to say, "There were never this many cases of childhood cancer, ADHD, allergies, and autoimmune disease."

Well, let's say that a lot of medical technologies aren't necessarily advances for health restoration. In fact, there's one technological advancement that was doing such a horrible job of injuring and harming people, the government had to step in. Vaccines. Except the government didn't step in to stop the program -- it stepped in to save it. Don't believe me? Keep reading.

> **A lot of medical technologies aren't necessarily advances for health restoration.**

In the 1950s, only four vaccines were commonly used in the United States. Smallpox and a combination of diphtheria, tetanus, and pertussis commonly known as DTP. In the decades to follow, there were several situations in which vaccines were causing harm and had to be pulled from the market.

Here it comes again, *But Doc, what about polio?* Well, based on the propaganda you hear today, polio seems like a miracle, even a hero of modern medicine. Think again. There is so much history and we could fill a whole separate book on that. The good news is that several really good ones have been written to tell that story.

In 1976, a swine flu epidemic seemed to be imminent. After four cases on a military base, President Ford launched the National Swine Flu Immunization Program. This program called for three steps. First, Congress was to allocate over $130 million dollars to produce a vaccine. Then, the government would handle distribution, and finally every American should get the vaccine. Sound familiar? Oh, one more thing, and this will be important to remember, the vaccine companies requested indemnity for any liability from any injuries caused by the vaccines. They didn't want to be responsible for the harm their product caused!

Beginning in October of that year, more than 40 million people got the swine flu shot. By December 16th, the program was suspended to investigate the serious side effects that were happening to some of the people who had received them. These side effects included hundreds of cases of paralysis and death. By March of 1977, the program was dead.[13,14]

Of course, this raised what some today still refer to as vaccine hesitancy. I do think you should hesitate, at least long enough to read the product insert, educate yourself, and decide for you and your family if this is the right course of action. If, after you do that, you still determine this is the right way to go, by all means, that is your decision to make. I've read the studies. I'm still hesitant. In fact, I'm going to hesitate forever.

I'm not the only hesitant one, though. Through the 1980s, a portion of the population became more hesitant. It didn't take long before the United States government washed away the risk of liability for vaccine injury. Vaccine manufacturers pushed for indemnification, threatening to leave the country without what was perceived to be almighty, life-saving vaccines. And key to many foreign policies. Again, another story.

In 1986, President Reagan signed the bill into law. The vaccine manufacturers carry no liability for any of the injuries they may cause.[15] There's no incentive to make a better product, they aren't liable!

Most parents today--and I'm talking a very high majority--don't understand the healthcare decisions they have the right to make. They believe they are absolutely required to give their children up to 36 doses of vaccines simply to go to their first few years of elementary school. From there, the annual check-ups continue ,and the push for more boosters and any new vaccines continue along with them.

Parents! You have the right to say, "No! I disagree! I will make the healthcare decisions for my family!" In almost every state, there is some form of exemption that is available for parents for their kids. But you have to educate yourself and be prepared to step in front of your children and say the word. In order to do so, you will likely have to read more than the simple, comforting, pastel sheet of paper handed to you. Ask for the product insert. Reclaim your position to make healthcare decisions for your family.

DARE TO DISAGREE!

I hope you are ticked off. I always tell my team there is one way to growth: Pain. Use the pain and anger you feel to disagree and choose health restoration and wellness for your family! It would be horrible if we ended there.

But there's good news! There are still doctors, nurses, chiropractors, acupuncturists, and other practitioners who have gone to those schools and have learned to think differently. They are still out there and getting amazing results and helping people to restore their health. This is why I take great pride in my Doctorate of Chiropractic degree! We were taught the principles vital to reducing stressors impacting health and how to support the body as it restores function.

What you're going to find in this book is a different way of thinking. A different perspective. This way of thinking is changing the lives of people across the country, giving them hope, and getting them results they never dreamed they could have. I hope you laugh, but you might cry, and you might even get upset – guess what? That's okay. Hang in there with me.

Standing up and saying, "I disagree," is the most powerful thing you can learn to do. It's not destructive. In fact, when done based on facts and not emotions, it can be the most constructive thing a person can do! Simply saying, "I disagree" can start a conversation that needs to happen. This book will show you why and how. I'm excited and grateful to bring you the information our clinics across the country share with their patients every day. Disagree with a thought process that doesn't work! Disagree with a healthcare system that is clearly broken! Disagree with shattered hope, take a stand, and think differently!

13 "The Swine Flu Immunization Program of 1976." Gerald R. Ford Presidential Library and museum. Accessed February 29, 2024. https://www.fordlibrarymuseum.gov/library/exhibits/swineflu/sf.asp.

14 Sencer, David J, and J Donald Millar. "Reflections on the 1976 Swine Flu Vaccination Program - Volume 12, Number 1-January 2006 - Emerging Infectious Diseases Journal - CDC." Centers for Disease Control and Prevention. Accessed February 29, 2024. https://wwwnc.cdc.gov/eid/article/12/1/05-1007_article.

15 "H.R.5546 - 99th Congress (1985-1986): National Childhood Vaccine ..." Congress.gov. Accessed March 1, 2024. https://www.congress.gov/bill/99th-congress/house-bill/5546.

CHAPTER 2

EVERYBODY HAS A STORY.

I love stories. They connect people and help them to understand each other and situations in ways that wouldn't happen otherwise. Everyone has a story. Every demographic, every walk of life. Regardless of who, or what, or when, what is common to all of us is that we each have a story. Our stories shape who we are and who we become. Together, our stories impact what happens in our generation today and in generations to come.

As you go through your life, you face circumstances and situations that change you. It's part of the process and essential in determining how you think and look at the world. Sometimes, you learn from things you go through yourself, and other times the experiences of others can have a tremendous effect because they share their story with you.

I'm going to share pieces of my story that have laid the groundwork for our family's legacy. I have learned from things I've gone through myself, as well as things I've watched others experience. It has all led to thinking differently. Thinking in a way that has empowered me and others to make lasting changes in their story. Changes that seemed impossible at times. Changes for the good.

This first story started when I met a girl that I fell in love with, and I fell hard! We knew mutual acquaintances who had tried to set us up on blind dates months before, but we had both bailed. I was busy with school, or at least that was my excuse. But over two decades ago, a chain of events occurred that would change my life forever. I will never forget the day I met her.

During the summer of 1999, I was a water skier for a show ski team from my hometown of Crivitz, Wisconsin. One day the pyramid fell on me, and I gashed my cheek. I also had a mild concussion, so I went to get adjusted by a chiropractic buddy I used to intern with. While I was there, a beautiful young lady with blond hair, short shorts, long legs, and platform heels came in without an appointment. We were introduced and hit it off immediately! I later learned this was the SAME girl

I was set up on blind dates with, the ones we had both bailed on. Crazy, right?

Two days later, we started dating. No joke! She told me, "I'm going to marry you someday," and I told her, "I think you're right!" There was something amazing and unique about this girl. We spent the first couple weeks of our relationship sharing our hearts and what we each wanted for our lives. She shared her dreams; I shared my vision and direction for my life. We discussed the family we wanted to have, where we wanted to live, our passions, and our goals. We also shared how we would raise our children and how we wanted to make a difference in the world. Remember, we were young. My career was just getting started. We had the whole world ahead of us.

Two weeks into our relationship, I went to her house, excited to see the beautiful woman I had fallen in love with. When I got there, she was sobbing. My first thought was, Uh-oh! What did I do, now? I thought things were going so well.

She had gotten her period that day, leaving her crying and in tremendous pain. She was always so happy; I had no idea she had so much pain in her life. There was more to this story than just female problems or hormone issues. In order to understand the bigger picture of what was really happening, let's step back a bit and look at Christy's life and health history.

Christy had struggled most of her life with various illnesses and conditions, and they got progressively worse as she entered college. Years later, she told me that before we met, she had never pictured her life past the age of twenty-five. That's how sick she was.

CHRISTY'S THOUGHTS

What was I thinking that day when Patrick found me sobbing and in pain?

Why would a guy like him—someone so confident, bold, and driven to achieve his future goals and dreams—want to be with a girl like me? You see, I was sick and had had many health challenges throughout my life up to that point. We had already talked about what we dreamed our futures would look like. I honestly didn't know what my future would look like, because doctors had given me a grim outlook. I had excruciating GI issues including ulcerative colitis that was on the road to becoming Crohn's. The medical doctor's best advice at the time was, "drink Maalox before and after every meal." Seriously? I did that, and I was so much worse! All they could offer me were more drugs and later on surgery would be inevitable. To me that was crazy!

Around that same time period (while I was in college), my reproductive issues also began to take over my life. From migraines to incredible cramping, I felt like every organ of my body was slowly shutting down. The doctors and specialists monitored my symptoms and then suggested drugs. I refused the drugs, so they insisted on monitoring me monthly with ultrasounds. They confirmed that I had cysts on my ovaries and that I had endometriosis. They told me I would probably not be able to bear children, or if I were to conceive, I would not be able to carry the pregnancy to term. Then they graciously offered to scrape my uterus. I politely said, 'no thank you,' and never returned to that office again. My mom had also shared other details of my health history, that I was a DES (diethylstilbestrol) baby. My mother was given DES shots while I was in utero to keep her from miscarrying me. But that drug is now known as the morning after pill. Quite the opposite effect. However, DES babies were discovered for having reproductive issues and damaged reproductive development which led to them having challenges getting or staying pregnant, or carrying pregnancies. As a result, I was at peace with the fact that I might not be able to bear my own children. I could definitely adopt some day.

So, getting back to this pivotal, emotional day, Christy began to share with me for the first time the health struggles that she had endured. I was shocked she was struggling like this; I had no idea. She even went so far as to say, "maybe we shouldn't be together." Now, I had a decision to make. While we had been sharing our hearts in those fantastic first two weeks of our relationship, I had shared with her that I wanted a big family. So, I had a choice to make right then and there. Do I stay with her, or do I leave her? I'm not kidding when I told you I had completely fallen head over heels for that beautiful woman. Do I chalk this up as a setback? Or do I choose to use it as a setup for one of the greatest gifts God has ever given me?

Because I loved Christy and we had a future in front of us that we both clearly wanted, the choice was obvious. The choice was her; it was us. It was easy to choose us because I had fallen madly in love. She asked, "But what about your dream of having children? The doctors say I might never be able to give you a child."

When I looked at that beautiful woman that I had fallen in love with, I realized that two words would define our future. I disagree. I disagreed with every doctor she saw. I disagreed with the general practitioners. I disagreed with the gynecologists. I disagreed with the specialists. I even disagreed with the chiropractor, who was giving her regular adjustments and great supplements. The beautiful woman I fell in love with was meant to have children just like every other woman. There was something they were all missing. I didn't know what it was, but I was determined to find out.

I obsessed in the study of female hormones. I devoured everything I could find, every research article, every study, everything. I spoke with other doctors I respected, people who had been my instructors while I was in school, and others who had a mindset to look at things differently than the doctors who were giving her no hope. I wanted to see multiple perspectives and put the pieces together. I studied female hormones like a fanatic. The best answers I found were disheartening. All I could think was, Man, this can't be all there is! I knew this didn't line up with what I had been taught in school. I couldn't settle for what I was finding. I knew there was more to it. I had to keep digging and look at it from a different approach. I had to think differently.

Just because we have what appears to be a fairytale life doesn't mean it was easy. We had obstacles. Every decision you make will have obstacles. The question is, will you overcome the obstacles to get to the end you want?

CHRISTY'S THOUGHTS

Some people say they wish they knew exactly what obstacles they would face in life so they could prepare. In my case, if I had known how hard my journey was going to be, I don't think I would've had enough courage to walk it. By the grace of God, I was introduced to a man I fell in love with and he turned my world upside down. For so long I felt alone in my health journey. Appointment after appointment I kept hearing the same two things: "We aren't sure why" and "here are some drugs and surgery to help your pain." I was discouraged to say the least -- even a bit depressed at times. The medical method was getting me nowhere, and I kept feeling worse. I couldn't eat typical healthy foods like salad, certain fruits and vegetables, and I had been allergic to dairy since the second grade. I had been seen and referred to so many doctors, but no one could give any answers on how to become healthy. I was exhausted and ready to try something different. So, imagine me on the floor crying, being vulnerable with Patrick for the first time. I was so afraid of what was going to come next. But then he said something that no one ever said to me before. "Don't worry about any of this. You're going to be okay." I chose at that very moment to trust him—a guy I just met—with my health and future. How crazy is THAT?!? I knew that this road was not going to be easy to travel, but the medical model had nothing to offer me that made sense. I chose to trust the process of the journey we were going to be walking together.

I may have been a new doctor, but I was convinced a woman's body was meant to have babies. My education taught me, and I firmly believe, all bodies are created for homeostasis. Homeostasis is health and function. That was more than any other doctor had offered her. I chose to look at things differently and not settle for the answers she had been given.
This unfamiliar approach was foreign to both of our families. As a result, it caused stress and struggles within our relationships.

We chose to stay with it no matter what, including all the criticisms that come when living under a microscope. What's the result? What was the impact of our decision to pursue Christy's health? We have four amazing daughters. Yes, I have FOUR daughters. You can please all pray for me now! I joke, but they are amazing and bring so much joy to our lives.

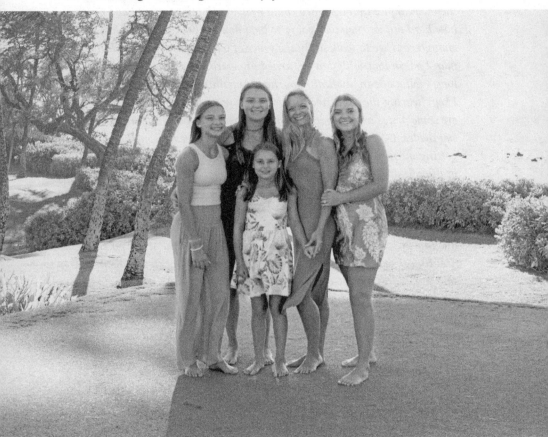

Sometimes I wonder what my life would have been like if I hadn't chosen Christy. If we hadn't disagreed with what Western medical thinking offered. I know it wouldn't be as amazing as life with Christy and these four girls.

There's another huge impact from that original choice to pursue a different understanding of health. One I hadn't known at the time when Christy and I chose to build a future together, a result impacting men, women, and children worldwide. It was a change of thought process. I had to look at things from a different perspective and not just settle for the "one size fits all" method the allopathic medical world uses. Now others are learning to ask questions, think differently, and even to disagree. That is a big deal for a culture that has historically never questioned anyone in a white coat; they are considered the experts. There is a lot of power in those two words, I disagree. More people are saying it because of the decisions my wife and I made as young, dating twenty-somethings. If you think about it, that is a significant impact. Much bigger than we could have imagined at that time.

Actually, a huge company, with clinics across the U.S. and a growing international impact, supporting countless people a year from around the world, would not exist if I hadn't chosen my wife. The Wellness Way wouldn't be where it is today if I hadn't chosen Christy and her unique health. This pivotal change of thought process impacted my wife and created the opportunity for us to have a family with those four amazing daughters. Now I'm using our experience to help families all over the world. I'm here to empower you in your choices; they have an impact. My impact all started with a change in my thought process. But I'm getting ahead of myself. Let me tell you about what I learned, and you can decide for yourself.

IS COMMON NORMAL?

I have some simple questions for you. Don't worry, I'll help you along with the answers. Would you agree in the past 30 years, we have more hospitals? That's obvious. More doctors? There's a specialist for everything! Spend more money on health care? We spend more on health care than ever before and our country spends more than any other country! Do we have more medications? Yes! The average American is on four to seven medications. We also have more medical interventions than ever before. With so much more medicine, you would think we would be the healthiest people on the planet. I had to keep reading and researching because I knew there had to be a better way.

The stuff I found was mind-blowing. For women, it seemed as though every life stage, literally everything her body is designed to do is seen as a condition that requires medical assistance. No wonder women are confused, struggling, and suffering! Let me ask you a question. If you have a daughter, when she gets to her teenage years, she's going to go through a change in life, correct? It's called puberty, and it's natural. It happens to every young woman. Yet, there are times when the evidence of puberty (the menstrual cycle) is inconvenient, so the medical approach looks for "solutions" to problems that don't exist. These are natural phases of life.

There was an interesting article I found in a very popular "health" magazine. It was all about the horse hormone given to young women to stop them from having a menstrual cycle. The article starts: "Sick of your period? Get rid of it!" I read the article and thought, maybe this is the thing, maybe they have it right. Actually, I didn't think that at all, but I had to read to see how they thought this might be a good idea.

At the University of Florida Health Sciences Medical School, with the assistance of medication, doctors have now agreed that cycles are optional.

But only with the help of medication. I started to research this idea further, and I found that doctors believe there is no medical reason to menstruate. Ever. I had to read what the medication does to make this possible because this obviously wasn't a natural process. The prescribed medication causes the uterine lining to harden, so you won't have a period anymore.

That sounds simple, however, physiologically, everything still needs to function as it was designed to. What do you think this causes the uterus to do? Like a balloon, it gets bigger and bigger until it actually explodes. The doctors agreed this is not dangerous; however, it may be inconvenient. I'm sure they have their reasoning for that thought, but ladies, if your uterus explodes, is that a little bit more than inconvenient?

I spent time reading thousands of articles by the best doctors in their field, and this was the best I could find. This was the only thing they had for my wife. How frustrating this must be for you ladies. After all my reading and research, after seeing hundreds of women a year in all stages of life, I can speak with great confidence about one thing. You want to know what it is? I thank God every day that I don't have a vagina. Every day. Guys, we are pretty lucky and have it pretty easy. We really do. I also started to realize women didn't understand their own bodies. My wife, at that time, was twenty-three years old and had no clue. Many women today have no clue what is going on with their bodies. They don't understand men and their hormones, and men don't understand their own hormones nor those of their partners. The medical treatment women are getting is a strong indicator that traditional thinking is failing all of us. I think it's time for all of us to look beyond what we may have been told. It's time for more people to disagree.

Think about some of the statistics we see daily. Now versus any time in history, do we have more or less heart disease? More or less cancer? More or less fertility problems? If we keep on that same thinking, most of you will have the same situations as everybody else. Just because something is common does not mean it's normal.

I wrote this book so that I can show you a different perspective. You need to think differently in order to get different results! See for yourself how I began to understand these hormones and functions and how we are able to convey this approach in offices all over the country. Not only are people thinking differently, but they're getting the clinical results they want and so desperately need. How are we doing this? That is what I and a growing group of doctors are calling The Wellness Way Approach. With the increase in medical advancement, should we really have more cancer, more infertility, more autoimmune issues, more heart disease, and more unhealthy people? Many people think because it is common that it's normal. By the end of this book, I want you to disagree.

A NOTE FROM CHRISTY
On being the first patient of The Hormone Whisperer:

I'm just a small-town country girl who fell in love with an amazing small-town guy. He had a vision in his heart to help people regain their health. I'm honored to have been his first patient in this way and to see where it has led. It's overwhelming to think I had some small part in that. I remember the day Patrick came to my place and I was on the floor in a fetal position. There were a lot of emotions.

I remember him just brushing it off when I told him I was probably not going to be able to have children. He said, "I disagree, don't worry." I figured we would cross that bridge when we got there. He was so sure, and I trusted in that.

Patrick was the only person willing to connect the dots for me. He was the only person who bothered to look for a solution. He gave me hope. I had learned enough to know I wanted to do things naturally. I was already under chiropractic care, but what I didn't know was the power of chiropractic care.

Many people only think of chiropractic care as pain management for physical trauma. There is a whole philosophy of chiropractic relating to the 3Ts (trauma, toxins, and thoughts) unknown to so many people. Once I understood where true health came from and how to regain homeostasis, there was no turning back. I met Patrick and I never stepped foot into another OB/GYN's office. That was it. I was all-in. I never looked back. He practiced adjusting on me. He took me to all his chiropractor friends who had graduated before him, I was adjusted by all of them, including doctors with whom he had interned. Patrick was determined to figure out why my body was so sick and to return it to normal. We both disagreed, and now he had to teach me how to think differently.

We did some dramatic things, such as completely eliminating sugar from our lives! I remember the day like it was yesterday. I cried. I was emotionally addicted. My mother and grandmother had taught me to bake. It was how we showed love and care for our family. I had to make a decision -- to be healthy or remain sick. Now, years later, I love to create new recipes using healthier ingredients comparable to those treats from long ago in the kitchens of my childhood. It's not easy. You have to make a choice. Treat everything you put into your mouth as either bringing life or bringing death.

Patrick proposed to me outside of a new hospital. I imagine this may not sound like the traditional engagement story, but it is a huge part of our story. We were walking the quiet path on the hospital grounds with the soft lights and large snowflakes falling around us. I didn't truly understand at that point. Can anyone really understand what is to come? It was romantic in our way. I understood his heart, his dreams, and vision. I knew as long as we would walk through it together, it would be worth it. He was proposing to the woman he loved in front of the paradigm and dogma he battled. He told me if I agreed to be with him for the rest of our lives, it would include a journey, an uphill battle. Patrick wanted me to know I was saying yes to not only him, but this life. I knew no matter how hard it would get or what adversities we faced, it would all be worth it.

When he proposed to me, did I have any inkling that our life would look anything like it does? No! Oh, my goodness, no! When I was a kid and dreamed of my life, I never dreamed past age 25. I would never dream about marriage or life past that point. Ironically, we got married when I was 25, and my life completely changed. I couldn't have pictured it if I tried.

In the beginning, this new life was a struggle. I lived on an island for many years, going against the grain. No one was doing what we were doing. As the years went by, we built a community of people, educating and inspiring them to become healthier and to create healthy families. We created the community we needed right in Green Bay, Wisconsin. The dynamics of our city changed. We had patients go to the grocery store requesting healthier ingredients, eliminating the need to have to drive to Milwaukee on a regular basis just to stock our pantries. This community of people who used to be sick and unhealthy became a transformative group of like-minded individuals. They were taking a stand for what was needed for their own health and their family's health.

When we were ready to start our family and stopped trying to "not get pregnant," I got pregnant right away. I was so excited. We told people right away. We didn't live in fear. We didn't seek the hospital route. Instead, we chose to have our sweet and precious babies at home with a midwife.

Don't allow someone to tell you it's not possible. Don't allow someone to try to scare you or make you believe lies. God created us to be mothers. We need to support and encourage each other. We need to reinforce this within a broken healthcare paradigm. There is a different way—The Wellness Way. This is the pathway to create a healthy family. We need to ask a different question to find the answers we need. What isn't functioning correctly? Why isn't it functioning correctly? Be willing to approach hurdles in a different way than you have before. You may be amazed at the people who come across your path who have the answers to the prayers you've prayed.

I'm excited for the many people who can be helped by this approach. This is about getting results. The principles and testing allow us to give people hope, answers, and the ability to see things differently. Patrick always talks about the importance of being able to step back and approach your challenges with a different mindset. The Wellness Way approach is an idea – an idea that says we are not genetically programmed for disease or illness, but for health. It's based on the philosophy that you can only truly be healthy if you address all 3Ts. We test because everyone is unique and should be treated that way. How are these 3Ts affecting you? They focus on who you are and what you need, not a standard procedure.

This book and the I Disagree seminar help people look at all healthcare options. If we could do that for one person, it has all been worth it. The best part is knowing so many people can be helped. After Patrick started helping me, women began coming from all over the place. They included a friend my age who was prescribed pre-menopausal drugs, to others who were given no choice but to take some form of artificial hormone. Word travels fast. Now women are calling from around the world. I've been able to watch as Patrick has been able to offer different answers to so many women. He's given hope to those who want to bear children, building their own legacy and future family, and impacting their children's children. Raising those healthy kids is another whole adventure! We are creating a healthier society, one baby and momma at a time.

Looking forward, I'm excited to create a different legacy of thought. I don't fear my girls not having babies. I'm excited. I talk to our girls about having children and a large family if they choose. It is joyous to discuss bringing life into the world and doing what God has called us to do as women. He's given us gifts to do what men cannot. The gift to be mothers. I want my girls to embrace it. To know that being a mother is a blessing. It's something to be celebrated and not treated as if it were a disease to be fixed or medicated.

I'm very proud of the man Patrick has become, and I'm excited to see how God continues to use him. I'm blessed to be on this journey with him and I can't imagine life without him. He's affected so many people, and I'm inspired not only by that man's brain, but also his heart. Of course he's good looking, but ultimately, talking with him, the way his brain works is so intriguing. I could listen to him teach all day. I wanted to marry an intelligent and intriguing man. I love learning from him and how we look at the future: learning, growing, and continuing this journey together. My husband never stops researching. He seeks out the best quality labs and products to ensure the greatest results in all the clinics across the country. The only variable is what you will choose.

ON THE "TO DO" LISTS

As he was coming up with the To Do Lists, Patrick started telling me about the things I was doing to help our marriage. I wasn't even aware that I was following a To Do List! Every once in a while, I'll gauge myself to make sure I'm keeping up with my end of the To Do Lists. Even though I helped to create them, I know I need to stay mindful to continue with them for our marriage. They can change a marriage. I know what marriage was like before the To Do Lists and the results once they are implemented. Every marriage has struggles but having useful tools helps point the way to a better marriage. Use the tools and the To Do Lists.

Both the husband and the wife need to come to a point where they are humble enough to recognize the needs of the other person. We need to recognize we don't have to be the same. Patrick and I are two totally different people. When you respect, recognize, celebrate, and embrace each other's differences, an amazing marriage can be built. When women complain, nag, or talk disrespectfully to their husbands, I just want to pull them aside and tell them they don't understand their husband.

They need to learn the art of listening to understand, instead of listening to respond. Likewise, a husband shouldn't be stressing his wife. He needs to stop trying to fix things we're just trying to share. He may not understand that he is causing her stress, and in doing so, depleting her hormones. It's a two-way street. If a husband and a wife can humble themselves and honestly look at what they need to change in their own behaviors and actions, it's a recipe for a better relationship. Listen, pause before responding, don't jump to a reaction, ask questions, be curious.

Ladies, your partner may not want to read the book, his hormones may not let him sit still that long! He will love the seminar. He will enjoy the entertaining approach. You'll leave with real tools to put to work right away. Get you and your husband to a seminar. Almost every woman who comes to the seminar without him tells us, "I wish I would have brought my husband!" If you are looking for answers or highly entertaining information, you'll find it at the I Disagree seminar. It's a fresh perspective and look at a topic that affects every man, woman, and family. Check in with your nearest Wellness Way clinic for the I Disagree seminar schedule on the Dr. Patrick Flynn website for details. It will change your life.

When a partner can gain insight into their marriage and what could be going on physiologically, new hope is born from hopelessness. This isn't just a story. This is the dedication and passion of our life. This is our real-life story. I believe it gives hope.

This man is the love of my life. He's the incredible father of our four beautiful girls. From daily dance parties when daddy gets home each night, to watching an occasional romantic "chick flick" with me snuggled on the couch – he always puts us first no matter how busy he gets.

CLOSING THOUGHTS

I love our story. I love that Patrick is so passionate about hormones and the irony that we have four girls! We have a new legacy of mommas. I'm thankful and grateful for what

God has given me: my husband, my children, and my part
of this story that has come to change so many people's lives.
It's overwhelming.

I'm on my knees daily praying for my husband and
The Wellness Way. We are on a quest to continue the relentless
pursuit of doing the right thing and getting the information
out to the people. We will continue regardless of what comes
our way, regardless of the hate mail and regardless of obstacles.
One of the biggest lessons I've learned and wish to pass
on to you, dear reader: Don't let your future be dictated by
someone else's fear.

CHAPTER 3

FIREMEN AND CARPENTERS.

My wife went to many practitioners before I met her. She saw obstetricians, gastrointestinal specialists, neurologists, chiropractors, a naturopath, and so many others in her search for help. They each had their own answers for her. The medical doctors prescribed drugs and suggested scraping out her uterus. She knew that wasn't her answer. Christy looked at the side effects and she knew she wanted a family one day. The natural doctors had her on a ton of supplements that cost her a lot of money. She was taking all of those supplements when I met her! She was trying to do everything right, but she still felt worse. She couldn't eat a salad because her digestion was so messed up. That's where she was when I found her crying in the fetal position on the first day of her period. How do you think she would have felt five years later? Or ten years later? She would have been very sick, because up until that point, her doctors had one mindset. That mindset is what keeps people from restoring function, what keeps them simply managing symptoms.

That is one of the worst feelings a person can have. To feel trapped by illness with only answers from the "experts" leaving you further trapped.

How many of you have sat in a doctor's office and been told that there is nothing they can do for you? Or what they can do for you is a drug with a bunch of side effects? You might have also been told that there is nothing wrong with you. Even though you have a laundry list of symptoms, they might not be able to give a diagnosis—so there is nothing they can do for you. That is one of the worst feelings a person can have. To feel trapped by illness with the only answers from the "experts" leaving you further trapped.

Anyone who knows me knows that I love to create analogies and use them frequently. Why? We've all sat with doctors, we made sure that we were listening, maybe even took notes. We even told them we understood what they were saying! Then we left the appointment and thought, what in the world did they say? The doctor sounded very smart but didn't connect with you. You had no clue what you were doing, and you were taking him or her on faith. I find analogies are much easier to remember than the language of doctor speak!

Do you know what many of them consider the best solution for addressing female hormone concerns? The best compound they had to develop a treatment for female hormones was horse urine. Seriously! I know, it sounds ludicrous; but it's true! Before I sit down with a woman, I go through the list of medications she is taking. If a woman is taking something like Premarin, I ask her if she has an affinity for carrots. Why do I ask her that? Most people don't know that Premarin comes from pregnant mare urine. It's a funny question, but I'm trying to get her to think differently. When they look at me confused, I say, "Well, you are putting horse urine into your body, and they like carrots and sugar cane, so I was just wondering."

Women are stunned when they learn what has really been prescribed to them. They should know, though. Would you agree that if a woman has been given a horse hormone and doesn't know it, she should be upset? Absolutely. I don't have a problem with someone taking something as long as they know what they are taking, what it is doing, why they are taking it, for how long they will be taking it, and all the effects that go along with that plan. Although let's be honest…how often is there a plan? Especially one that works toward getting someone off a prescription. That's not how that system works.

Let me share the analogy that has set the foundation for everything since I started. It sets the basis for every patient that we work with. If you understand this simple analogy, you will understand there are two very different systems and which doctor to use for which situation.

Some of you are reading this book because you are frustrated with your doctor. Especially now that you have started to change your thinking. This is something I want to make sure you read closely. I'm not saying you shouldn't go back; I'm saying you should know why and when to go back. By the time we are done here, I want you to be able to have a clearer understanding of health and be confident in your choices. I want you to know when to say, "I disagree," and when to let them save your life.

FIREMEN AND CARPENTERS

Let's say you've been out for a nice evening with your family, but you get home and find your house on fire. Who is the best professional to manage this emergency? That seems obvious, but follow me for a minute. The fireman has the best training to handle the situation.

So, let's walk through the scenario. The fire truck pulls up, and the firemen have two primary tools to work with: hoses and axes. The firefighters run up to your house with their axes.

Even though they caused massive destruction, you are not mad.

They crash your door in and smash the windows. Next, they start spraying the inside of your home with their hoses. When the water they spray hits your family photos, what does it do to them? The wall? The carpet? The fire department has been there for about fifteen minutes, and what have they done to your house? While it isn't livable anymore, you are grateful for the many ways they have destroyed your home!

All you have left is a burned-out shell and you are grateful. Even though they have caused massive destruction, you aren't mad. Why? Because they did their job! Can you live in that house? No. Is it toxic? Yes. Could it kill you? Possibly! Remember, the fire department did an excellent job and did everything they were supposed to do with the knowledge and tools they had to work with. But that doesn't mean your house is fit to live in.

44

Eventually, you'll want to get back into your house and continue on with life. Who is the best professional to call for that task? The carpenter. Imagine if the carpenter shows up while the fire department is still there. The carpenter sees a mess! He has to rip out walls and carpets and bring in the materials he needs to rebuild the house. Which person is right? Both, based on the specific need of the house at the specific time. If the carpenter shows up to the house while it's on fire, what good would he do? Now you might laugh at this question because it's so obvious, but it illustrates my point! If he shows up with his tools of a hammer, nails, and lumber, he looks like an idiot! Vice versa, if the fire department shows up and tries to rebuild the house with an ax and a hose, you would think the guy is crazy. Would you agree? Based on the need, you have to know which professional to call.

If you understand that example, you understand how healthcare should be run today. If you are having a stroke or heart attack, would you trust me with the education I have to run into your kitchen and grab a knife and see if I can help you? No! We need to call someone who is the best professional to save your life. Who would you prefer we call? We should call 9-1-1.

For the purposes of the analogy, let's call traditional medicine the fire department. They're going to take you to the hospital and use their axes and hoses on you. Here's where some confusion comes in. When they put the hose into your arm and start pumping the medicine into your body, is it good for your body? Some say yes, and some say no. Let's go back to the example. When the fire department sprays water on the walls, is it good for the walls? You have to answer the question that was asked. I didn't ask if it saved your life. I didn't ask if it put out the fire. I asked if it was good for your body. If you look at the back of the medication bottle and the inserts, there are numerous warnings and negative side effects, and they are definitely not good for your body. The manufacturer presents this information. I'm not saying the medication is not needed, I'm just asking if it's good for you.

Now, let's say the medication didn't work. They only have one other tool: the ax. Could you possibly die from that surgery? Okay, can we come to an agreement? Could we agree that if you are having a heart attack, you may need drugs or surgery to stay alive? Even if they aren't necessarily good for your body, they are what is needed at the time to save the body from dying.

Can you rebuild a house with an ax and a hose? No, you can only put out a fire.

Let's go back to my wife. Did they give her medications when she presented her symptoms? As the fire department, they start with medication because it's the tools they have to help her. The challenges my wife was dealing with would eventually develop into cancer. Then it would be time for the ax. They would tell her to have her uterus removed via hysterectomy. She went to some top specialists, but their way of thinking was still the fire department philosophy. Do you follow me?

Let's look at another example. Can you guess the number one reason why people have gone to the doctors in recent years? High blood pressure. Everybody knows someone with high blood pressure. Can someone die from high blood pressure? Yes! Do I have any problem with the fire department's approach using ACE inhibitors, channel blockers or Lasix? No, they have the potential to save people's lives.

But after the life has been saved, after all the warm thank-yous to the doctors and nurses, do they ever sit down with you and discuss why you've had the heart attack or stroke? Do they help you get your body back to healthy function? They may suggest a bland diet and an occasional walk, but are they helping you to rebuild for a long and vibrant life? Can you rebuild a house with an ax and a hose? No, you can only put out a fire. Can you get your body back to normal with drugs or surgery?

No, you can't. You can only manipulate the body to adapt to a stimulus or suppressant.

Today, we have many fire department doctors. We need them in certain instances! But we also need carpenters. The Wellness Way Approach is the carpenter approach. I want to know what triggered your fire. We help our patients to repair the weak spots where fires can start, rebuild where fires have been, and, best of all, find indicators of possible future fires before they happen so that you can live that long and vibrant life!

When Christy presented me with these problems, I figured out what triggered her fires and how to rebuild her house. That's why we have our four daughters today.

Let's take a look at another example in my office. What's the number one medication given for high blood pressure today? Many people take the medication Atenolol. And although this drug can save a life, let's not forget one of the negative side effects listed is extreme fatigue.

I had a woman come in with female hormone problems as well as extreme fatigue and thought I could help her. I looked at her medication list and told her I couldn't help her unless I found what was causing her to have high blood pressure. If I didn't

> **The key comes back to finding the trigger.**

find the cause, she could never remove this medication which was causing the fatigue! Do you see the difference in thought process? The firefighter approach would have put her on something to change her energy level, correct? Could that have worked? Yes, but now you've added another medication. If you watch TV or read ads in magazines, you will see medications competing over who can put out the fire faster. But they missed the point. I ask a different question: What caused the fire in the first place? The key comes back to finding the cause of the dysfunction.

THE STORY BEFORE THE STORY

I met my wife when I was almost done with chiropractic school, but some of this story started even before that. You are probably assuming based on my success that I come from a wealthy family and was loved by all my teachers. That's not the case.

Shortly after I married Christy, we ran into one of my old teachers at the grocery store. She didn't tell Christy that I was her favorite student. As I stood with my new bride by the frozen meats, my former teacher looked her dead in the eye and said, "I never thought he would become a doctor. I thought he'd end up in prison." My new wife looked at me with eyes that said, "What did I get myself into?"

I came from a hardworking family that worked to make the best for their children with what they had. My mom worked in a bank and had a second job as a waitress. My dad was a truck driver. I know that I was a hard child to raise and give them credit for doing all they could do. I was hypersensitive, my skin was always crawling, and I could never sit still. When the teacher had us work on a writing project, I was drawing a picture of myself hunting on the back. It was always a very elaborate drawing, but I got a zero on that homework. I loved hunting, and I couldn't focus on the project my teacher wanted me to do. As the years went on it got worse. My mind was going a mile a minute. I could not sit still. Today mainstream medicine would have diagnosed me with ADHD and had me on a bunch of different drugs.

I see that today in my practice; they want to put children on drugs. I learned to think differently early on and now I can help kids who are going through what I went through. I know now that the body doesn't always need drugs, especially if we remove the factor that is causing the problem. I discovered I have an egg allergy that was triggering my system. If someone had looked at what was happening to my body and understood the approach I use now with my patients, it would have been a lot easier on my family. It would have been a lot easier on me. But I wouldn't be who I am today, which is someone who thinks differently.

WE ARE NOT THE SAME!

A lot of people think because we think differently than the traditional medical approach that we are the natural approach. They get so excited when they see me. "Hey Doc, I totally get it. I don't take any medications and want to do things all natural." I reply, "Hold the phone. You're taking twenty supplements! What happens if you don't take those supplements?" They say, "Well, I can't poop." If you need to take a bunch of supplements to poop or feel normal, then you're still sick. You're still sick because the thinking of the popular natural movement and mainstream medicine are the same. We have to change that thinking.

The natural movement will apply the same medical thinking to your symptoms but with natural remedies.

The body doesn't make mistakes.

The system of medicine leans toward acute care or treating the immediate problem or symptom. We call them firemen because they put out your immediate fire without addressing the rebuilding of the body. The natural approach has taken on that same thinking. Instead of giving you an ACE inhibitor for your high blood pressure, they treat your symptoms with fish oils, B12 shots, CoQ10, magnesium, potassium, and other natural remedies. They are treating the symptoms instead of finding out why the body is displaying the symptoms. One patient can have high blood pressure for a totally different reason than another.

This is where the principles of chiropractic teach another perspective. The body doesn't make mistakes. If there is a symptom, there is a reason why the body is trying to adapt. It's not the symptom that you need to fix. You need to test and find out how to get your body to function. We are all so unique that we can't rely on the standards of care the allopathic model of medicine applies to every person as if they had the same physiology! If you think of your neighbors, family members, or your spouse, everybody is different. Why would applying the same medication or natural treatment to every body benefit everyone? It wouldn't. That's why it's important to test to find out what is happening with the body. It doesn't make any sense to assume everybody needs the same thing and that just because it works for one person, it will work for everyone with those symptoms.

There is one guy who is famous for this in the natural realm. Dr. Oz! He could put a one-armed man on his show and give him turmeric and somehow, miraculously, his arm grows back. When his arm grows back, what happens with three million one-armed men the next day? They go out and buy turmeric. Boy, are they disappointed when their arms don't grow back. This is called the Dr. Oz Effect. I didn't make it up. Google it. It's a real thing! Not the arm growing back, the Dr. Oz Effect.

The Dr. Oz Effect is what happens when a product or treatment is featured on his show and tons of people rush out to try that product. The challenge is all these people are unique and have different reasons for their symptoms. The Neti Pot was featured on the Dr. Oz Show and sales went up dramatically! The increase in people searching for info on the Neti Pot was even more astounding. Nobody ever searched raspberry ketones and green tea extract, but after mentions on the Dr. Oz Show, they were trending. The "King of Natural Remedies" always has something new to offer, and people rush to try it.

I hear the strangest things when I travel and do seminars. Some of the craziest are from some people who you'd think might know better, most of those are people trained as natural health practitioners. "At least with the natural movement, you don't get the side effects of the medical system." She stumped me there for a bit, she was right. After a lot of thinking, I thought of one side effect—a smaller pocketbook.

You'll spend all that money on supplements, but what will you get for it?

I want you to think about something, which will fail first, the medicine or the natural option? The thing about treating symptoms with natural remedies is that they will fail when compared to a pharmaceutical drug. A drug can force your body to do something. If you give a guy Viagra, his body will respond whether he wants it to or not. That doesn't happen with natural methods. Have you guys heard this about natural remedies, or had it happen to you? You took something, and it helped for a little while, but then it stopped working. It didn't continue to work like it did in the beginning. It gives you false hope, and then you're back on the medication you were on in the first place because you never restored function, you tried to use a natural substance to act like a drug. The good news is that they don't work that way. They are created to support, not manipulate. But the method of supporting here is all wrong. It's being used to manage symptoms, not supporting the body to restore function.

CHRISTY'S THOUGHTS

Before I met Patrick, I had tried just about everything. When I started to take some homeopathic tinctures and herbs, I felt a little better, but months and even years later I was still struggling with the same things; and if I didn't take my supplements—man, was I in excruciating pain! I'm sure there are many women who can relate to what I am saying. Anyone can push a certain product on you to try. At the end of the day, you need to ask how is this really making me healthier? It didn't make a difference what I took because I was asking the wrong questions. Instead of asking what can I take to make me healthy, I should have been asking what is not functioning? Where is my body deficient? How toxic am I?

That's why the natural mindset movement and the Dr. Oz Effect are failing people. They take the same approach as the medical system, but it doesn't heal the body. It may (or may not) mask the symptoms for a while, with a natural product instead of a pharmaceutical, but it doesn't get to addressing the body as a whole. That's why The Wellness Way Approach is different. We aren't the medical approach and we aren't the natural approach. We think differently.

I didn't just balance my wife's hormones to get her pregnant four times, I got her body healthy.

I tested my wife from a different mindset. I looked at what triggered her fire and asked, how do I rebuild her body? I didn't just balance my wife's hormones to get her pregnant four times, I got her body healthy. It's perfectly normal for a healthy woman to have a baby. That's a positive side effect! We don't test for fires, we test for what could trigger a fire and how to rebuild the house in such a way as to prevent that fire from ever occurring again. I know you didn't pick up this book to read about hormone issues. You really didn't. You were looking for something else, something that seems elusive. It's not. Stay with me. Let's talk about health and how we got here.

CHAPTER 4

WHAT IS HEALTH?

At my seminars, I ask people to raise their hand if they want to be healthy. When I look out at the crowd, I know they all want it. No matter what their job is or how big their house is, they all desire health over illness. They want it for more than themselves; they want healthy kids, healthy parents, and healthy in-laws. Okay, maybe not that last one, but you do for the rest! Just kidding.

The funny thing is, for as many people that want it, very few people can tell me what "health" is. I hear a variety of answers and even a few responses of "I don't know" when I ask them to define it. You would think for as necessary to life as health is, most people should be able to offer an acceptable definition. Unfortunately, we've only been taught how to manage sickness and symptoms, not to restore health.

We've been taught about fires our whole lives. Fires like cancer, diabetes, heart disease, and all the others you see in drug commercials. Everybody wants to be healthy, but we know very little about it. How can you have something, or even want something, if you don't know what it is? That's why so many people are sick today.

Here's another question I ask people: What are three things that make you healthy?

I already know what they will say. We've been conditioned to think specific things make us healthy. Every audience answers the same way:

Food, exercise, and sleep.

I hear these answers every time. Just about everyone in the audience agrees. Unfortunately, it's yet another reason why people are so sick. These three things have very little to do with making you healthy. You know people who never eat well, never exercise, smoke every day and live to be a ripe old age. George Burns lived to be 100 and we all know that he was very open with his cigars and martinis. Then you have people who simply come in contact with second-hand smoke and get lung cancer. Ladies, you know you hate those women who eat four donuts in the morning, never exercise, and are thin. Why are they healthy even though they are eating unhealthy things and not exercising? But are they really healthy, or just thin? There's a difference!

You may be confused now and think I believe that food, exercise, and sleep aren't important for you. I didn't say that. I asked you if that is where health comes from. They are very important to your health, but they aren't where health comes from. Just like when we talked about the house on fire, is putting the water on the walls good for the walls? We need to start thinking differently.

Let me give you an example from my office. I had a nurse practitioner from a local hospital visit me. She thought she had some hormone problems. We went through our normal exam, where I took some x-rays and saw a tumor. You know what I told her to do? I told her to go back to the hospital and check to make sure she wasn't going to die. Why? Can I rebuild the house if you are dead? No.

They took a biopsy and decided since it wasn't going to grow so they'd just monitor it each year. That was the decision between her and her fire department-type doctor.

Let's say it was cancer and could have killed her. If they pulled it out, did they extend her life? Possibly. Did they make her healthy? No. According to statistics, within two to five years she would very likely find herself with a new tumor. When you tell people from the "natural" side of healthcare the reason we live so long today is medicine, they tend to freak out. Drugs and surgery have done a good job of

> **Drugs and surgery have done a good job of keeping us alive. But, we are still sick as dogs because they don't make us healthy.**

keeping us alive. They are doing their job. But we are still sick as dogs because they don't make us *healthy*.

Earlier, I explained how definitions are important so that we can be on the same page and know what to expect. I don't like the definition of health that suggests as long as we are just being kept alive or surviving a condition and treating symptoms that we are healthy. Those are two very different ways of living. So, I created one that I think is more accurate. Here's the definition of health we use at The Wellness Way:

health [helth]

noun a condition of wholeness in which all the organs are functioning 100% of the time.

If I cut my finger and my body is functioning well, it will heal. If my body is not functioning well, there are conditions where I could bleed to death. Let's go back to the three healthy choices of food, exercise, and sleep. If I cut my finger, do I have to eat a healthy salad for it to heal? Do I have to take a nap? Jump on a treadmill? Funny, but do you see the difference? Those choices are good to help rebuild your house, but that is not where health comes from. Health is about function.

Remember our definition of health? *A condition of wholeness in which all the organs are functioning 100% of the time.* Our body is designed for *homeostasis*.

The definition for homeostasis is very familiar in the chiropractic world: *A self-regulating process by which biological systems tend to maintain stability while adjusting conditions that are optimal for survival. If homeostasis is successful, life continues. If unsuccessful, disaster or death ensues. The stability attained is actually a dynamic equilibrium, in which continuous change occurs yet relatively uniform conditions prevail.*

That's why people who do unhealthy things are still healthy because their bodies don't get pulled out of homeostasis.

Homeostasis is the scientific word, but all it really means is balance, or normal function. For some of you, this balance is simply between health and disease, but there is more to it. The body has three states: normal function, adaptation, and disease. There is an ebb and flow within those states. Your body was built for normal function, and that is the best place for it to be. Oftentimes we spend a lot of time in the adaptation state before

> **Your body was built for normal function, and that is the best place for it to be.**

moving to the disease state. Generally, people are unaware of these three states and where exactly they are existing. Nobody worries about it until they reach the disease state. They don't worry about it because their body is doing all the work to adapt and maintain life.

Adaptation is the state between normal function and where symptoms show up. You can be in this state for a long time and not know it unless you're properly tested. It is in the disease state that we see those fires. Let's say your hormone levels are really high. Your body has left homeostasis and is in the adaptation state. If it stays there a long time, it will likely move to the disease state. The same happens if your hormones are really low. Your body is in the adaptation state; if it stays there long enough, it will likely move into the disease state. That can be said for any situation that indicates your body has been knocked out of homeostasis.

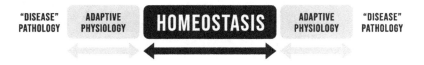

The reason why people are so sick today is because they jump back and forth between the states of adaptation and disease, rarely landing back in normal function. Our entire medical system reflects this. If your M.D. runs a test, they're going to be testing for disease and treating your symptoms. Your tests look fine until one day, you have cancer. Then they treat your disease with a drug, but you stay in a state of adaptation that leads to dysfunction. Because proper function isn't restored, it's only a matter of time before the disease resurfaces.

The only way to stop the cycle between adaptation and disease is to find out what is triggering the body and remove that stress, that disruption, so the body can return to balance or homeostasis.

One thing that sets The Wellness Way Approach apart is how we view the body as a collective whole. If you present

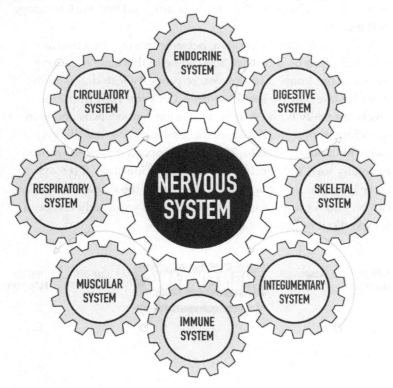

one symptom, it may be reflective of a health challenge in a seemingly unrelated part of the body. However, we know there are no unrelated organs or systems within the body. Everything is connected like an intricate Swiss watch.

THE SWISS WATCH PRINCIPLE

If you remove the back from a Swiss watch, you will see a bunch of gears. Some are large, and some are small. Some move fast while others move slowly. They all have a specific function for the watch to keep time properly. Imagine that the smallest gear stops working or breaks a tooth and no longer works correctly. What happens? The whole watch stops working efficiently and can't keep time accurately. Each and every gear needs to function properly for the watch to operate as intended.

The body is just like that. It is extraordinarily complex and composed of many parts. Did you know that your big toe controls

> # Did you know your big toe controls your heart? Yes, really.

your heart? If you smash your toe, what happens to your heart rate? It increases. Why? Because even that little gear can affect everything from your heart rate to your cholesterol. That's why it is important to look at multiple gears and functions. If you are experiencing symptoms with your heart, they might be coming from another system or organ (gears). You can't just treat the heart with medication. It could be a completely different gear that is causing that symptom. Keep in mind that medications have side effects that affect other gears. Adjusting and fixing the broken gear will help prevent unnecessary damage to other systems.

Have you ever known someone who took a medication for heart issues and later discovered it damaged their liver? Because the human body has so many organs and systems working together in harmony, you cannot treat one system (gear) without affecting others.

Detoxification is an important function, but it is only one gear. The gears of proper nutrition, structural care (what most people consider chiropractic when they limit that practice to simply physically adjusting the body), mental health (including proper handling of stress), and hormone function also need consideration. If one gear is not working properly, you cannot be healthy. Just like a Swiss watch, all need to function together.

If a person receives regular chiropractic adjustments but eats fast food all the time and manages stress poorly, they will not be able to achieve complete health. Likewise, if a person takes care of proper nutrition and detoxification yet neglects their mental health, they will never fully restore health and homeostasis. True health is when all the gears work together in harmony—this is complete health.

> **We address the cause (or causes) of ill health, not just the symptoms.**

The Wellness Way looks at each individual patient as a unique person. Clinically, we look at all the gears as a whole, just like the Swiss watch. That's why neither the medical nor the natural approach will work long-term without applying principles of health restoration. We have to find out which gear is stressed and how. One stressed gear could be the gastrointestinal system. As we know, the GI can affect many things, but so can the liver, the pancreas, and the heart. We look for which organ is stressed to see how it could be causing a cascade of problems throughout the body. We address the cause (or causes) of ill health, not just the symptoms. We don't just look at one gear; we look at the whole watch.

You just learned about one of the core foundational principles I work from each day. When a patient comes into a Wellness Way office with a concern, they have probably been seeing doctors for years who have run tests and couldn't find a problem. Those doctors did what they could, but they didn't look at the hormones, the gut, or other systems in the body that could be contributing factors to the current condition they are dealing with. They were looking at one gear. They needed to look at the whole watch.

ERIN'S STORY

My family started seeing Dr. Patrick at The Wellness Way when two of our three daughters had adverse reactions to childhood vaccines. We were super strict with the kids' care, but were certainly not as disciplined ourselves. After all, we weren't having seizures like our kids were.

Two years later, I noticed a lump in my breast. I was 32 years old. The first thing I did was call The Wellness Way. I was able to see Dr. Patrick immediately. To say I was anxious is an understatement, but we had found this fantastic community and knew it would be okay. When you walk in the door, you know you are in good hands. While I was meeting with Dr. Patrick, one of the front desk associates took two of my young daughters, so I could have a focused discussion. The first thing Dr. Patrick did was help me calm down. After an exam, he had me schedule an appointment with my OB/GYN to order focused testing. He assured me he was confident I would be told the cyst was benign. He said they would likely suggest just watching it over the next several years. Dr. Patrick went on to ask a few more questions. By the time I left that first appointment, I felt much more confident.

The next appointment with my OB/GYN went as Dr. Patrick predicted. She did a quick breast exam and ordered additional tests. During that time of waiting for appointments, our family had other visits with Dr. Patrick. Each time he would give me pieces of information to research. He already knew what I was going to face and wanted to prepare me. His confidence calmed me and my husband immeasurably.

Immediately after the appointments and initial rounds of testing with my OB/GYN, I was taken for additional testing. After a few days, I received a phone call. I was told the cyst was benign and they would keep an eye on it. I went back to Dr. Patrick armed with my good news. His answer was simple. I was "safe" for now, but my estrogen levels were abnormally high. I had a choice to make. I could either let things go, and in 3-5 years, I'd most likely be facing a cancer diagnosis with 3 young daughters and a husband in my mid-thirties. Or I could work to get healthy now. It was an easy decision. Let's do this and get healthy! The date was October 17.

Dr. Patrick laid out the plan for me. I would have a very restricted diet for six months, and the first few weeks would be especially intense. At the end of six months, I'd feel like a whole different woman. I was also excited at the prospect of losing the extra 40 pounds I was carrying. I had recently met a young woman about my age at church who had won her battle with breast cancer. I asked her what she knew about estrogen-fed cysts and breast cancer. She pointed at her now flat chest and hair freshly grown back and told me she wished she had known more.

Remember that restricted diet and the date? The very next day was my daughter's birthday. I chose to give her a healthy momma and not have a piece of cake; and for the daughter who had a birthday two weeks later; and the next daughter, 3 days after the second. I said "no" to unhealthy eating at Thanksgiving, Christmas, and all the holiday gatherings, including New Year's, Valentine's Day, my husband's birthday, and our wedding anniversary. Finally, six months later, on my birthday, I was able to indulge in a piece of fruit. Dr. Patrick was and is right. Food is emotional. Your health is largely dictated by the eating choices you make.

I had a lot of questions from family and friends. I didn't want sympathy. I didn't need critics. This was an intentional decision to give my children a healthy mother, my husband a healthy wife, and to reclaim my health. I cut out all sugar and nearly all my favorite foods. I learned a lesson that would affect many decisions we would make for health in the coming years. I was able to teach my beautiful daughters what has now become a family mantra – "food is fuel, not a friend." Was it hard? Yes! Was it worth it? Undoubtedly.

I've not been back to the OB/GYN since. Why? The cyst dissolved, I lost 40 pounds that haven't come back in nearly 15 years, and as a woman in the second half of my 40s, I know what a big deal both of those situations are! Had I followed their advice, I wouldn't be where I am today. My husband may have been a single father with three young daughters. I didn't want to play their guess-and-wait game. There was too much at stake. For any woman wondering if taking care of herself and/or her hormones are worth it – absolutely. Look at your children, look at your husband. Get over the "hard" and do the hard and right thing. There's too much life to live. Choose to live it.

CHAPTER 5

STRESSORS.

Chiropractors help the body deal with stress. This puts them in a unique position to look at health differently. I learned about dealing with stress well before becoming a chiropractor, including the beginning of my adventure to Palmer Chiropractic College. Stress happens. It's how we deal with it that can make or break our health.

I was finishing up my last semester at the University of Wisconsin–Green Bay and had sent my transcripts off to Palmer Chiropractic College, where I'd be going to school in October. It was June, and there were just days left until final exams, when I got a call from the admissions office. They said I was missing a class. I said, "I'm not missing any classes. I have them all." They said, "Oh wait, you have an exercise physiology class, but that doesn't count as a physiology class."

I said, "That was a 300-level physiology class, and I was told that would be approved. I start there in October! I'm not going to wait another semester to start for a physiology class that I took." My mind and heart were racing.

They said, "Listen, we have a community college here that offers that course. You can finish it in six weeks. Then you can start school early." I had a choice to make either start in July or start in February. I asked when the class started. The next Monday! I was a twenty-two-year-old guy in Green Bay, Wisconsin, on Tuesday, with exams to finish. The class would start in Iowa on Monday, I didn't have much money and had nowhere to live. What did I do?

I scrambled. I finished my exams on Friday. I found a room to rent in a house with upper-level chiropractic students. My parents and I packed their pick-up and headed to Iowa. I made it down there in time to take the course I needed. I made it happen.

I went home six weeks later to visit the weekend before I officially started at Palmer Chiropractic College. Bad luck struck again on my way back to Iowa. I was in Illinois, twenty miles from the Iowa border, when my car died. I couldn't get it started, so I tried to flag someone down. No one would pull over.

Finally, this college kid heading to St. Ambrose University in the same town stops. He said he'd drive me to that far, but I'd have to find a ride from there. I hopped in. When we got there, it was the middle of the night. There was no ride to be found, so I walked six miles to my new house with all that I could carry. I was stressed about how I was going to tow and fix my car, but I had class in the morning. Moral of the story? Stress is everywhere. We encounter it every day. It's how you deal with it that matters.

CHIROPRACTIC IS ABOUT ALL STRESS. THE 3T'S!

Some people say I'm "just a chiropractor" in a demeaning way, but I'm proud of the potential of chiropractic care. Many people believe chiropractors are just pain doctors, or for after accidents. Unfortunately, through some of the regulations and restrictions that have been put in place, you read about those in Chapter 1, and some creative marketing, many people agree with that perspective. Well, I disagree. I'm proud of what I can do.

> **Some people say I'm just a chiropractor, but I'm proud of the potential of chiropractic.**

Chiropractic helps me look at things differently. Through studying chiropractic, I learned what stresses are and how they impact the body. Once you know and understand that you have the philosophy and insights to help remove them and allow the body to heal.

What damages our health? What knocks our body out of homeostasis? Stress, or what we call the 3Ts in chiropractic.

Traumas, toxins, and thoughts damage our health. These are the 3Ts that chiropractic was meant to address at its foundation. Unfortunately, due to a wide variety of reasons, chiropractic has gotten away from its original directive. This means the value of what chiropractic can do is being overlooked.

66

The 3Ts are the stresses that disrupt homeostasis. Stress is a stimulus that can produce mental or physiological reactions that may lead to illness. Technically speaking, stress is a disruption to homeostasis which may be triggered by internal or external functions or experiences.

Common thought is that chiropractors are in the best position to help with physical stress or trauma. What does a chiropractor do? Remove physical stress. You may be thinking, no, Doc, my chiropractor makes my pain go away. Have you ever gotten adjusted, and the pain did not go away? Let me raise my hand first. Have you ever gotten adjusted, and your headache did not go away? Let me raise my hand first.

Today the fire department medical system so dominates the way we think, we define all professionals from that perspective. That's not how chiropractic works, though. We've been taught chiropractors do just one thing. They are the carpenter doctor who removes that physical stress. But typically, that's not the only stress. There are other stresses our bodies are exposed to because of our choices. If the body has a symptom, it is adapting to a stressor. We can find out what that stress (toxin, trauma, or thought) is and remove it.

To really understand how to keep the body in balance, we must understand each of the 3Ts.

WHAT IS TRAUMA?

Chiropractic has a different definition of trauma than typical mainstream culture. In chiropractic, trauma is defined as anything that puts the body under physical

> **Your body doesn't make mistakes. It responds to stressors.**

stress. This is what most people think of when they think of a chiropractor.

If I run at you and attack you, what is going to happen to your heart rate? It goes up. What is going to happen to your blood sugar? It goes up. What happens to your cholesterol level? It goes up. Are you seeing a trend here? If we draw your blood at that moment, what will medical and natural doctors think? They will look at the results and say you are sick, or you need intervention like a drug, therapy, or a supplement. What is your body really doing? It is responding to physical stress on your body. Your body doesn't make mistakes; it responds to stressors.

Remember that big toe example? If I smash your toe, what happens to your heart rate? It goes up. Blood pressure? It goes up. Sugar? It goes up. Cholesterol? It goes up. That is physical trauma. Your body will adapt to the physical trauma it encounters daily. No matter who you are, your body encounters trauma. Heck, your body encountered trauma coming into the world through the birth process. Don't try to tell me you don't have any physical trauma!

That's why when people say that they don't need to get adjusted or their kid doesn't need to get adjusted, I respond, "Wait…. you're telling me your child has no chance of physical trauma? Did your child learn to walk? Did they fall? Does she ever cross her legs? Does he ever lift things incorrectly?" See what I'm saying? When you remove that trauma, you leave room for the body to heal. All chiropractic really does is remove that physical trauma so the body can adapt. The body just wants to heal and return to proper function.

Let me give you another example. Let's say your plane was rerouted from Hawaii to Green Bay, Wisconsin during winter. You packed for summer, not the frigid temps of the frozen tundra. If you went outside in shorts and a tank top, you would be pretty cold. What would happen if you stayed out there in negative temperatures for a long time? Your body would send all the blood to your core to protect the vital organs. That is an adaptation of the body. But, if you stayed out there long enough, could you lose your fingers and toes? Yes. The body didn't make a mistake. It tried to adapt to the stressors and kept you alive. It was your choice to walk outside and stay out there.

Your body always makes the right choices and adapts, even when you don't.

Speaking of choices, our modern, fast-paced, quick and easy lives mean we make a lot of choices that expose us to toxins.

WHAT ARE TOXINS?

When I was a kid, my grandpa owned a bar across the street from our house. Every day, I would go across the street, open the fridge, and grab a Coke. Then he'd give me a Kit Kat. To this day, sometimes I still want a Coke and a Kit Kat. No matter how healthy I eat, the memories associated with those foods still create cravings. I know now these food choices are just one example of the many toxins our bodies encounter every day.

> **Toxin exposure begins in your mother's uterus.**

Toxin exposure begins in your mother's uterus. Her toxins became our toxins as they traveled through the placenta, however, it didn't stop there. When you were born, you were most likely vaccinated and injected with toxins. Toxins like lead in paint and toys, prescription drugs, beauty products, soaps, shampoos, artificial air fresheners, and cleaning products. Even if you have reduced your exposure by being careful not to use toxic products, and eat super healthy foods, toxins are still in the air you breathe and water you drink.

Toxins are inflammatory foods like sugar, dairy, and wheat. And surprisingly, even really healthy, clean, organic foods can be toxins if you are allergic to them! It is so hard to avoid all toxins, of course. All you can do is eliminate all that you can and support your body to take care of the rest.

I know what you are thinking …but Doc, our bodies naturally detoxify. That's true, the body is built to detoxify. But, our bodies can only handle so much before it becomes difficult for the body to naturally detoxify. Toxins build up when the detoxification mechanisms cannot keep up with the production of cellular wastes, or the absorption of toxins from the intestines. In other words, garbage is coming in at a faster rate than your body can process it and safely remove it. Those toxins build up, and when your body can't adapt anymore, can knock you out of homeostasis and make you very sick.

Exposure to xenoestrogens is very common in today's modern society. To make it simple, let's call this chemical "estrogen." Xenoestrogens are a subcategory of chemical endocrine disruptors that have an estrogen-like effect. What do you think it does to the body's homeostasis if you are throwing in a bunch of fake estrogens? These chemicals are everywhere. BPA, phthalates, and parabens are common xenoestrogens. They are in plastics, household cleaning products, dryer sheets, cookware, food, and beauty products. These are products people come in contact with every day. They are causing disruption and are building up in the body of a high percentage of the population.

There are environmental toxins that we may be unaware of or can't control in the air or water. Mold can be toxic for many people. It is a hidden killer that can cause inflammation, hormone imbalance, and immune system issues. Chronic exposure can be hard to identify because it messes with the body in so many ways. The toxicity suppresses the immune system, which can trigger other illnesses. And since finding the source often means relocation if their home is the source, many are unable to eliminate the source or believe they can't afford to. In reality, they can't afford not to. People look at their symptoms and the illness and don't always connect them to mold sickness. In the long term, this can lead to even more serious illnesses like cancer or autoimmune disorders.

You're not sick. Your body is trying to adapt.

Many people don't connect the dots between the toxins that are causing the disruption and their symptoms because the effect doesn't seem immediate. In other cases, the reaction can be swift and clearly connected.

If I give you a shot of gasoline to drink, what will happen to your blood pressure? It will go up. You are probably going to puke, run a fever, and get diarrhea. Your body is adapting to the toxin. You're not sick, in fact, that is a healthy reaction! Your body is trying to adapt. It's trying to bring everything back to homeostasis. You may have been the one who made the bad choice to drink gasoline, but your body is making positive choices so it can adapt.

All illness or condition is a long-term adaptation for survival. We look at things that stress the body and go from there. When we assess a patient, we look for what is stressing the body. Imagine if I stressed you out like crazy, and then you went for a check-up at the medical doctor immediately after. They are going to tell you, "Your blood pressure is high. Let's inhibit and stimulate the body to a normal level." They'll use drug or surgery interventions. What an incomplete way of looking at the situation! Did they ever look at what was causing the high blood pressure in the first place? Wouldn't it make more sense to look at what is triggering the stress and remove that?

That's why understanding toxins and detoxification is so important. We will talk about that more later. There's another "T" that we have to discuss, and this one is a big one in today's society.

WHAT ARE THOUGHTS?

This is the stress most people think about when they think of stress! It's the mental stress that I encountered when I started chiropractic school. It's the mental stress that you encounter every day. It's huge! Most people don't realize the impact it makes. Now, don't get stressed out about your stress just yet.

First, let's start with who stresses out more, men or women? Women. Who causes women the most stress? This is where my audiences laugh and call out, "Men!" Guess what—they're right! I'll prove to you that men are one of the biggest contributors to illness on the planet today. I'm not joking!

We are up at night stressing about our stress. It's a never-ending cycle!

Hang with me though, guys, it gets better.

Every day we are bombarded with worries like bills, work, getting kids to school, health, household chores, and all the expectations to keep all these things afloat. Then we find out how bad stress is for us and stress out about that! That means we are up at night stressing about our stress. It's a never-ending cycle!

It's important to reduce stress because it can impact every system in your body, and when one system gets out of whack, so can others. Remember the Swiss Watch Principle? For example, when stress puts our body into the fight or flight mode it can impact our digestive system, and your body won't be able to digest the food you ate properly. This can lead to acid reflux, colon problems, hormone problems, high blood pressure, and so much more.

CHRISTY'S THOUGHTS

That pivotal day that Patrick found me—you see, I get it now. When Patrick told me, "Don't worry, you will be okay," he was removing one of my stressors without me realizing it. He knew that I was depleting my hormones worrying about my health and future. So, when I hear friends or some of our patients frustrated about the length of time that the healing process takes, I just need to say that I UNDERSTAND! My biggest piece of advice: Trust the process! As a patient, you need to step back, follow the guidance of a Wellness Way doctor, and stop stressing yourself out! All you are doing is prolonging your healing process. I did not get well overnight. It took many years of continuous baby steps in the right direction and Patrick asking different questions in order to come up with different solutions to what I was going through. If you hit a plateau in your healing process, don't stop or give up! Keep going! Wellness Way care is about peeling back the layers and discovering the next area that needs focus. Many times, a breakthrough is just around the corner!

Mental stress can make you very sick, especially if you are a woman. It is the biggest reason I see patients in my clinic. Mental stress can really impact a woman's health starting with her hormones. I want you to think about this. You can get adjusted and pull all the chemicals out of your body and eat organic but guess what is ten times more disruptive to health than anything else. Mental stress. It can lead to conditions that have the potential to kill you. All doctors are taught this. I started to study women and why they stressed out so much. I polled women eighteen years ago and I still ask them today, "What do women care about?" EVERYTHING. But what are the top three things that cause the most stress?

WOMEN

1. MEN
2. KIDS
3. WEIGHT

MEN

1. WORK
2. SEX
3. KIDS

Here's where I may surprise some women. Women, it's very clear where we are on your stress list. Ladies, where are you on our stress list? You're not. There's only one way you can stress out a guy, ladies. I'm going to show you there's a biological reason why in a few chapters if you will be patient with me. The rewards for your health and relationships will be worth it!

Some people might call these men workaholic, perverted pigs. I disagree, and if you stick with me, for the next few chapters, you will find out why there is this biological difference. It all comes down to hormones. Stresses impact all of us.

Understanding the 3Ts helps us understand how to mitigate that stress so that we can find and maintain homeostasis.

Most of us know common stressors to our bodies. That's when people get caught up in the idea of moderation. You know the phrase, "Everything's okay in moderation!" I disagree. Most grandmas are fans of moderation. You can also swap out for mom, dad, aunt, uncle, or any other person who has influenced the way you think about food, including grandpas who give you a Coke and a Kit Kat bar just for crossing the street.

Grandma has misled you on some things. You may be thinking, Doc, are you saying my grandma was wrong? Well, grandmas are right about a lot of things—and we love them dearly—but in their quest to spoil us, they often encourage some unhealthy habits.

Grandma has misled you on a few things

Let me explain. Grandma comes to you after you've started to eat healthy. She brings a plate of chocolate chip cookies with all the unhealthy, highly processed ingredients, and she says, "Here honey, I have some cookies for you," and you say, "No thank you, Grandma, I'm not going to eat those." And Grandma says, "Everything is good in moderation!" Grandma loves you, but her perspective is wrong.

I disagree with the concept of moderation. Your body doesn't know if something is good or not. It knows if something is inflammatory and creates stress or if it provides nourishment. It doesn't know moderation. It doesn't stop the inflammation process just because you only eat that food once in a while.

Eating is one of the most emotional things we do. Let me give you an example. Let's say I gave some health advice to a married couple; don't have sex for a week. Now the guy will be kinda mad, the gal will be just fine. Right? But here's another angle. If I tell that same couple to fast for three days, they'll both hate me. Food carries a lot of emotional influence. To help understand this point, I've defined moderation for us:

Moderation is your emotional justification to eat something bad for you.

It's just emotional, that's all it is. In the end, it all boils down to your choices.

Your body responds to your choices, regardless of whether they are good or not. So, you say, "Oh, come on, it's just one cookie!" But the body still has to do what? Adapt to your choices. Is not getting a regular chiropractic adjustment a bad habit? Yes, it is, so your body is going to adapt to not getting adjusted. If you eat a bunch of processed sugar cookies, your body adapts. If you are mentally stressed out about your in-laws visiting, your body has to adapt to it. Picture yourself getting away from people stressing you out and locking yourself in a room for an hour. What happens to your blood pressure? It goes back to normal. Blood sugar? It goes back to normal. Cholesterol? It goes back to normal. What stresses out the body? Trauma, toxins, and thoughts. Your body will respond and adapt according to those stressors.

Do we respond to the symptoms, or do we respond to the triggers?

That's how disease develops. Do we respond to the symptoms, or do we respond to the triggers? It seems pretty simple to me. Where it gets a little more complicated is that there is usually more than one stressor, and people respond to triggers uniquely. This is especially true if we are looking at the differences between a man and a woman. In this politically correct world, we don't talk about stresses the way they need to be talked about. Men and women are different. Yes, men and women need to be valued equally; however, in that argument, we must understand that valuing them equally does not mean they are the same. We need to be able to appreciate and empower both to be who they are in their masculinity and femininity, along with their biological differences. For our health and our relationships, this is absolutely necessary.

PART 2

HORMONES ARE THE
MESSENGERS OF LIFE.

CHAPTER 6

DON'T KILL THE MESSENGER.

Men and women are different. That doesn't mean one is of less value than the other. It just means they are biologically different. I don't try to make women something they're not, and I hope the women in my life don't try to make me into something I'm not. It would be a difficult task though—my testosterone is high, which makes me confident in who I am. You'll learn more about how this works later. For now, we need to understand that it is not only okay but necessary for women and men to be recognized as fundamentally different.

We live in a time when many people in society are saying we (men and women) should be treated the same. In terms of equal respect and dignity, absolutely! In terms of how we are created to function, absolutely not!

It's not because I'm a male or a chauvinist; it's because what they are saying doesn't make any clinical sense. When it comes down to it, we are confusing people. We are treating every person the same, and it's leading to sickness. All these women are coming in sick as can be, and it's the same for the guys. Why are so many people sick? Because they don't understand who they are or how they are biologically designed. We got away from understanding the differences between the sexes somewhere in the midst of trying to make them equal. So, to the idea that men and women are able to function in the same ways, I disagree!

Now for those ladies who are getting uncomfortable about this, please, let's slow down a bit and hear me out. I never once said you are weaker.

You can have a baby. I can't. You're nurturing. I'm not. You dominate in a lot of areas that guys can't. Equality can't happen simply because we're not equal. However, valuing each other for our individual gifts and what we can bring to the table is possible. We can't be like you and you can't be like us.

Here's an example: if a woman has a sex drive like a man, she is very likely going to end up sick, maybe even with cancer. Why? Because that woman has high testosterone, which isn't normal for a woman. If a woman has a sex drive every day, then clinically, I'm out of my mind worried about her. I want to get her tested to find out what is triggering her hormones out of balance. It's a signal that she likely has PCOS or some testosterone-dominant condition. It's biologically impossible for a lady to be healthy and dominated by male hormone levels, her physiology simply doesn't allow it.

Have you ever seen little boys and girls play together? They get along just fine. Their hormones are quite similar and consistent. Then, that magical time called puberty comes about and turns the whole relationship upside down. They don't know if they love each other or hate each other. Throwing two cats in a burlap sack would be more peaceful than watching two pubescent adolescents of the opposite sex try to interact. What happened? They still have the same genes and phenotypes, but something has changed, and it's changed dramatically. Their hormones have started to change their childhood bodies into the bodies of a man and a woman. They may not be able to describe or explain it, but they can sure feel it—and so can everyone else around them!

We have gotten away from the biology -- the actual science -- that in any other debate would be looked at as gospel. Biologically, I will prove to you beyond a scientific doubt there is no way a man and woman can think the same. Of course, they can agree, but that's not what we're talking about. I'm saying they aren't actually thinking the same way. It's physically impossible! There is just no way. Here, I can prove it to you guys.

> **It's biologically impossible for a lady to be healthy *and* masculine, the hormones simply don't allow it.**

Let's say I inject your wife with synthetic hormones. I guarantee, no matter which hormone, within a week she, will think differently. Do you know why? Because it will alter her brain. The same thing if we take a guy and inject him with a ton of testosterone. He's going to think differently very quickly. Do you want to know why? Lots of testosterone is going to affect his brain, also. Ladies, you know this. Your hormones change throughout the month. Your mental pattern changes throughout the month. It's a good thing for a normal functioning body. Don't feel bad about it. It is what your body was born to do! Men's and women's hormones are designed to make us function differently. Actually, to function in a complementary way.

Hormones are what make us who we are. It's what makes a man a man and a woman a woman. We are so dramatically biologically different, but we are trying to force men to be women and women to be men. And now, as a result, we are seeing consequences in their health.

What's tragic is that this goes beyond health and impacts our relationships. There are two things I see all over the country: very sick men and women and very disappointed men and women. Whether we realize it or not, our health can play a significant role in our relationships. Divorce is on the rise, and so are cancer, depression, and chronic illness. Could there be a reason or correlation? Maybe, just maybe, men and women need to understand why they are different and accept that as normal.

Maybe, just maybe, men and women need to understand why they are different.

I started speaking about this all from the physical aspect, but it became so much more when I heard from people whose health was improving. Women would say, "Hey Doc, I'm psychologically better and more in love with my husband, my marriage is so much better." Men would come up to me all excited, "I have a better sex drive and energy levels. My marriage is better!" That's how my original *Hormone Connection* seminar got started.

As patients started to see healthy results, they also had really positive side effects. How incredible is that? Marriages were being saved! When they started to get physically healthy, their mentality changed, which resulted in their relationships getting better. When you learn and apply this information, it changes your thinking. Once you change your thinking, we are ten steps closer to changing your health.

One night after a seminar, a man came up to me and said, "I wish I would have known this forty years ago. I would have treated my wife differently." That's huge! When both men and women understand the concepts I teach, a relationship can change direction. Here's the key: You have to understand how hormones work. They will dictate the physical and mental

> **Once you change your thinking, we are 10 steps closer to changing your health.**

aspects of the body. Don't believe me? Keep reading and let me prove it to you!

Even though we highly recommend bringing your spouse to the I Disagree seminar, one of the most frequent comments I always hear from women after a seminar is, "I wish my husband would have been here to hear this, too!" When both spouses are on the same page, it makes caring for their health so much easier. When a patient comes into my office, I prefer to meet with both halves of the couple. It makes the most sense. When both partners hear the message from the same source, there will be less confusion, and we will be able to communicate more clearly. Also, it will help the person we are most focusing on to have a support person. Often there are

> **Understanding those who are different helps us understand ourselves even more.**

real and practical steps the support person can do to help our patient. That's why I've written this book as if I'm speaking to both men and women, even though I know that women make approximately 95% of the healthcare decisions.

If the wife gets this approach and she shares it with her husband, and he participates, they will start an amazing process of getting healthy and having a happier marriage together. But wait—I'm not excluding you singles out there. This book is still for you! You can learn more about yourself and learn about others too. It's handy to know about both sexes in work and life. Understanding those who are different helps us understand ourselves even better. After all, knowing someone and understanding someone are two totally different things.

So, let's start breaking this down. In my seminars, I often ask women what they want in a man. I hear things like: Compassionate, kind, a good listener, thoughtful, gentle.

Ladies, I think I may have found the problem. You aren't looking for a man. What you just described sounds like another woman! When you understand the basic biological differences in our hormones, you understand the simple fact remains that men and women are very different at their core. No matter what media and Hollywood would have us think today, we aren't the same, and it has little to do with the clothes we prefer to wear. A man can't be a woman, and a woman can't be a man. There will be so much less angst in this world once we get over the notion of "gender confusion."

Remember when I talked about how easy it was for kids to play together before puberty? That's because during childhood, their hormone levels are roughly the same. So, let's say a child hits puberty and their sex hormones haven't regulated properly due to disruption or interference somewhere in the body. This could result in what some label 'gender confusion'—this means they are likely sick and need to have their hormones tested! They aren't the opposite gender trapped in the wrong body; their hormones are likely off from optimal levels and not communicating with the rest of the body properly.

To understand the difference between the sexes, we must understand hormones. What is a hormone? It's a group of specialized chemical messengers that make up the endocrine system. Each hormone has a special message. A hormone doesn't really do anything on its own. It's released by a gland like the pituitary, ovary, or testicle. That hormone goes to another cell and tells it what to do. But it doesn't really do anything other than act as a communicator. Then it breaks down and gets reabsorbed. A hormone is simply a chemical messenger. When people say, "I'm crabby. My hormones are off." What does that mean? It means the messenger is off. You know that saying, "Don't blame the messenger?"

Don't blame the messenger if something is off in your body. It's not the messenger's fault that something is triggering stress in your body. It's just telling the body the message it was given by the glands as to how the body can adapt. If the adrenals are stressed, that will impact the messenger. This can happen in all areas of your body, impacting various messengers that help the different systems of the body function. Everything from digestion to reproduction or thinking to growth.

> **A hormone is just a chemical messenger.**

Men and women have different glands and different messengers. Don't blame me for biology! I'm just the messenger here. This isn't my opinion. It's the physiological makeup of males and females. We need to really get into hormones to understand how they make us different. Since guys are the simplest, we are going to talk about them first. Once we figure out men, it will be a lot easier to understand women. You thought it was hard? This guy figured it out, and if I can, so can you! So, what makes a guy tick? Keep reading.

CHAPTER 7

WHY IS HE SO CONFIDENT?

Why am I so confident? Because I have made sure the primary source of my testosterone is optimized and fully functioning! I'm talking about testicles. Ninety-five to ninety-seven percent of testosterone production for a man happens in those glands. The other 3-5% happens in the adrenals. Testosterone is what makes a man who he is, but there is so much that goes into it. Once you understand the body like a Swiss watch, you understand that you can't just add testosterone to make a man. If a man has low testosterone, it's not that he is getting old or that his testicles aren't working. Let me explain to you how testosterone is made. It will help explain a lot. You'll understand why men have the traits that make them men and confident about it.

> **Testosterone is what makes a man who he is, but there is much more that goes into it.**

It all starts in the brain. Ladies, later, I'll give you a little insight on how to understand and communicate with the guy's brain in the way that will help you both. We're about to get into some biology and physiology; I'm not going to overcomplicate this. Just stick with me. The pituitary gland, or what we call the "master gland," is a little gland in the brain. This is where testosterone production starts. The things that happen in the brain can have an effect on testosterone or any hormone's production. The pituitary gland gets feedback from the hypothalamus (a specific part of the brain). The hypothalamus will release a gonadotropin releasing hormone that tells the pituitary to create follicle stimulating hormone (FSH) and luteinizing hormone (LH). LH is the big producer of testosterone. LH is the hormone that goes down to the testicle and binds to a cell. If LH isn't normal, you can't have testosterone. It starts in the pituitary; that's why it's called the master gland; it's what controls the functions of many of the endocrine glands. LH travels in the bloodstream down to the testicle.

The testicles are actually a casing for a half mile of tubules, cells put together, that are misleadingly called balls. Some of those cells are Leydig cells. Those Leydig cells have little receptors; those receptors are looking for LH hormone. Those Leydig cells need LH to be stimulated to work. That's the next stage of testosterone production.

The next factor for proper testosterone production is LDL, or cholesterol. I know most of you are probably thinking, LDL is bad! No! It's not bad. It's needed by the body for homeostasis. We will talk more about that later. The only thing you need to start the production of testosterone is LH and LDL (LDL is produced by the liver). Remember what we know about the body, it operates like a Swiss watch. What's happening in the brain and the liver can impact testosterone. The liver converts hormones and regulates the balance of your sex hormones. If something is off in the brain or the liver, your hormones can be way off. It's not just the testicle. The body is a combination of massive moving parts. To think everything has to do with just the testicle is incorrect. You can't just add testosterone and fix everything. Anything that disrupts the brain, or the hypothalamus, can disrupt LH production, which can disrupt testosterone production.

Testosterone is responsible for the physical and mental differences between men and women. It gives us energy, it gives us muscle development, and it gives us our sexual drive. Remember, hormones also change us mentally. Testosterone gives a man great confidence. Every healthy man, regardless of his age, thinks he's amazing. Right, ladies? Do you ever see your husband in front of a mirror? He's flexing and checkin' himself out. It doesn't matter how old he is. Testosterone gives us this great confidence! Ladies, you don't have the amount of testosterone we do, so you tend to downplay it.

When a man can be confident and unashamed, that's normal and healthy. Don't put him down for his confidence – encourage that boy! The second function of testosterone is to keep him motivated and driven. Testosterone is why he does what he does; it is a very driving hormone.

If somebody were to break into your house tonight, which of you would get up to chase the criminal? Your man will. Why? Because when testosterone rises, it makes him aggressive. That's not bad, unless it is focused in an unhealthy, uncontrolled way. Remember the big steroid hormone craze of the 80s? It was a craze, alright. What happens when you give a man synthetic testosterone to supplement his natural testosterone? He can go crazy with aggression.

Think about it. Who commits the most violent crimes, men or women? There isn't even a comparison. Men commit three times as many

> **Testosterone is why he does what he does.**

violent crimes as women. I don't intend to create an argument— those are the facts. Does that mean you should hate men? With that fact in mind, does it mean police hate men? No, it does not mean police are targeting men. Why, then, are men committing more violent crimes? If the testosterone gets too high from steroids or another physiological adaptation like a tumor, it can cause a man to commit a violent crime. It's one of the side effects of steroid drugs. Does that give men an excuse? No! Men need to be able to control that drive and harness it for good. Is this the only cause for violent crimes? Of course not, but it can most certainly be a contributing factor.

The testosterone range for women is generally between 5 and 40 Ng/dL depending on their cycle and stage of life. Men's range between 350-1200 Ng/dL. Even a guy at the lowest end of his range is more than seven times higher than a woman at the highest end of her range. A healthy man will likely be more aggressive and competitive than a woman simply based on his physiology. Recently there have been more crimes committed by women who are also taking synthetic testosterone. It is literally changing how they function toward this aggressive, more male trait. This idea that we can be mentally or biologically the same is simply untrue and causing harmful results.

Now some of you might have examples of men who don't have high confidence or motivation. These stories are all too common. But remember, common does not mean normal.

"Doc, my husband sits on the couch a lot more lately, but overall he's a healthy guy," says a woman in my office, there to take care of her hormonal health. My response? Oh no, he's not healthy! You know what her other complaint was? He isn't interested in sex. Does that sound healthy to you? It sounds like he has low testosterone to me. Ladies, if your husband isn't interested in sex every day, it's a sign his testosterone has been affected by some factor. Before that final signal happens, you may notice he loses his spark to get stuff done. This

Four out of ten men experience hypogonadism, which is another name for low testosterone.

guy is not alone. Four out of ten men experience hypogonadism, which is another name for low testosterone. Despite what the medical community has told you, low testosterone is not a natural part of aging. Remember, common is not normal.

This woman was sitting in my office because her hormones were off, but she didn't notice the signs that there was something wrong with her husband's main hormone. When women have symptoms of imbalanced hormones, they know what's causing it. They might think there is nothing they can do about it, but they know what is to blame. When a man's main hormone is off, there are mental factors that many will just brush off.

Most men don't get their testosterone tested until they are older and experiencing physical symptoms. Testosterone impacts a man's health, sperm production, bone mass, muscle mass, sex drive, energy, facial hair, self-confidence, and more. Low testosterone can lead to major health problems, including cancer. We want it to be at good levels.

What people don't know is most men will experience more mental problems before the physical problems manifest. Let me say that again. Men will go through more mental changes than physical changes when their testosterone drops down. So, when you see your man getting lazy and demotivated, it's an early sign something is going in the wrong direction.

What could be going on? In rare cases, it can be a tumor, but most of the time, it is because of unhealthy habits. If a young man has unhealthy habits as he ages, his testosterone will go down. It's not because he's aging! It's because of his unhealthy habits, including all the sugar he may be eating.

> **Whether it's a man or a woman, if their hormones are off, they will end up very sick.**

We dismiss it as aging, but it's not normal for an aging man to have their testosterone drop down. Clinically, Wellness Way doctors, including myself, could show you men in their eighties who have high testosterone. Testosterone levels are independent of age. Ask my wife. You can ask a healthy male. Ask a woman who has a healthy male. You know what they say about the healthy male? That boy is always going. My wife will tell you that I'm a healthy male!

You need to get your man tested. Low testosterone is not normal. Just like PMS is not normal, menopause symptoms are not normal, endometriosis is not normal, or any of the other hormonal conditions that we relate to women. It's one of my most popular quotes for a reason... common is not normal. Women and men need to take care of their hormonal balance throughout their life.

CHRISTY'S THOUGHTS

Yes, no doubt about it—my husband is a healthy male! It's the confidence and boldness that attracted me to him in the first place. I admit that early in our dating and marriage I didn't understand some of those masculine traits, but now I do and have come to embrace them in my husband. I don't want to change him. Testosterone traits define a man. God molds and defines his character. I am very aware of men that I encounter who are very obviously sick and don't even realize it, sadly, until their marriages begin to fall apart. Ladies, get the men in your life tested!! Learn to love the God-given qualities that testosterone gives a man, your man, and you will transform your relationship!

A healthy testosterone range is wide, but you want to see good, high testosterone levels. Personally, I want to see mine stay over 500 Ng/dL. One of the major things to watch for ladies is if your boy is starting to get lazy. It's not because of feelings. Testosterone is not impacted by feelings. If he has high testosterone, he is going to be on the move.

Trust me, testosterone will make the body do things. Don't believe me? Look under the covers in the morning. If your boy has high testosterone, you will see evidence of the testosterone salute. Testosterone is highest in the morning and fluctuates throughout the day. Morning erections exist regardless of how a man feels. Don't make your man feel bad about this–that's a sign of a healthy boy! His normal physiology will make him get an erection in the morning. Why? As those testosterone levels come up...so does he. It's independent of how he feels.

Ladies, most of you are attracted to a strong, motivated man. You aren't looking for a wimpy, demotivated man. Guys know this! That's why testosterone is so important to a man. This aggressive hormone makes us who we are. This is how biochemistry works. You want a feminized man? Let his testosterone come down. But trust me, you don't want that—it's not a good thing for him. When a guy sees himself, or women see the men in their lives (husbands, sons, fathers) becoming demotivated, it's time to make some changes. Most importantly, have him tested properly! Socially, we also need a new approach to how we see and appreciate guys.

CHAPTER 8

MEN ARE SIMPLE.

"Doc, my relationship with my husband has gotten so much better. The spark is back in our marriage!" I have heard this so many times, especially when I first started out in practice. I didn't start out talking about hormones and relationships. I

He can't control the rise in testosterone.

started out talking about how to help remove the stressors and restore proper function in the body. What my patients and I found out was that being healthy improves relationships. Understanding hormones improves relationships. I was just a doctor trying to give my patients the best functioning version of themselves. Better relationships were a happy side effect.

Here's one piece of relationship advice you can both thank me for. Imagine you've just had what I like to call a passionate conversation, some may call it a fight. Ladies, your hormones make you want to talk. Don't talk to him. His testosterone is too high; leave him alone. He'll cool off and come back with a much more level head and be able to have the conversation you want to have. Many devastating and mean things are said by husbands when they are mad. When he relaxes, that testosterone returns to normal, and you are both able to speak calmly, he always says, "Honey, I didn't mean it that way." And he didn't. He was responding to the rise in testosterone due to the rise in tensions in the situation.

He can't control the rise in testosterone. I'm not saying he shouldn't control his response—he absolutely should— but when people understand testosterone, they can have much more success during conflict. When his testosterone rises, it tells him to attack whatever is sitting in front of him. In no way am I justifying the horrific domestic abuse caused by disgusting men who are out of control. That reaction must be controlled. I'm explaining what a rapid rise of testosterone does in the brain.

Testosterone also makes him very single-task-focused. Once you realize where it comes from, it's very obvious to see it in various ways throughout his life. Ladies, your guy can only think about one thing at a time. Consider how quickly guys tend to climb any ladder of success. Men are driven because they can focus on just one thing at a time. Testosterone tells the guy's brain to go after whatever he sees. Think about that fact in terms of relationships. Ladies, do you think testosterone tells a guy:

"be nice to the girl" "romance the girl" "get her flowers"

NO! It tells him to "chase the girl!" See, often women want us guys to be softer, dare I say, more feminine. But we don't have the same hormones you do, so we can't be like you. It doesn't make us any better or worse than you, it simply makes us men. What most likely attracted you to that guy was that his hormones were complimentary to yours. He pursued you with a clear purpose and was relentless in that pursuit. In the evening, a man's testosterone starts to decrease a little bit. His ability to listen and focus increases. He's also more agreeable, passive, and low-key. Ladies, let me tell you step one in how to win with your man. If you try to tell your husband to do something in the morning— you might as well have not told him at all. Let me give you an example.

> **If you want to talk to your man and have his focused attention, don't do it in the morning!**

You ask him to take out the garbage. He's laser-focused on the day ahead of him. He's not really listening to you, and he leaves. When he closes the door and walks out, the garbage is still left there. Upset that he didn't listen and help, you begin to stress. During the day, you imagine all the possible reasons why he didn't take out the garbage. We've all been there. On his side, he's forgotten about it the minute he left the door! Testosterone has him so focused he's in his own world. He didn't hear you, but you stew all day, either mad or with hurt feelings. You end up creating a lot of stress and can even make yourself sick due to the reasons you've created in your mind before having a conversation with him.

When he comes home, he has been laser-focused, energetic, and aggressive all day and you've been imagining things and frustrated all day. Your first response is to question why he didn't take out the garbage like you so sweetly asked him that morning. His response is, "You didn't ask!" and you're off to the races with another fight. Ladies, understand if you want to talk to your man and have his focused attention, don't do it in the morning. This will save so many fights. If his testosterone is normal, he's already in high gear and not hearing you. I know some call this selective hearing. He's really not trying to ignore you; his brain is just flooded with the morning dose of testosterone he naturally needs to make it through the day.

CHRISTY'S THOUGHTS

I'm going to be honest, real, and vulnerable with you. I made plenty of mistakes early in our marriage due to not understanding what testosterone did and how to keep my man healthy. No one teaches you about hormones or how our bodies are supposed to work and act, so how are we supposed to know what to do when things start to go wrong? To top that off, most people have never learned how to set healthy boundaries either. As I walked my rocky journey of becoming healthier, I realized that as my physical health began to improve, my mental health needed to change too. You see, when a person grows up dealing with constant health issues, a 'victim mentality' can emerge, and when I realized that some of my words, thoughts, and actions were not healthy, I had a choice to make. I could keep thinking the same old thoughts, speaking the same old destructive words, and doing the same old bad emotional habits, or I could choose to THINK DIFFERENTLY.

I chose and still choose to this day to examine myself daily and make changes when I see they don't line up with the priorities I have set in my life. Think of it this way—if you have a pebble in your shoe and walk on it all day long, what is your mood like? Probably irritable and perhaps overreactive, right? Well, if you remove the pebble, but don't address how you react to things, you may unintentionally be hurting others with the way you speak or respond to them. So, as you are healing physically, don't forget to take the time to do the 'hard stuff' of getting brutally honest with yourself and healing emotionally as well.

THE MAN ZONE

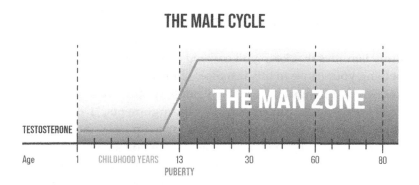

We've discussed the fact testosterone rises drastically during puberty and remains high his whole life. I want your man in the Man Zone all the time, that's normal.

What do you think is the most common challenge with men in the Man Zone? I hear ladies say (as if it's a bad thing), "But Doc, you don't understand, my husband wants sex every day!" My response is simple. That's a good, healthy boy! Are guys perverted? Are they disgusting? Nope. Sexually driven? Yes. And guess what. Men, that's part of being a man. Be proud of it! Women, you married him because you wanted a man. That's part of the package. Now remember, just because he wants it every day doesn't mean he gets it whenever he wants. A woman always has a choice, and men have to do their homework.

I do want those guys to stay in the Man Zone. If they don't, they'll get very sick. I'm going to teach you, ladies, how to build his testosterone and keep your man healthy. You can help him increase his testosterone, so you can get him to do virtually anything you want. I'm going to give you a To Do List. Don't worry, I'm not putting all the work on you. You get off easy. The men will have two To Do Lists. Trust me, they can handle it. They have testosterone to motivate them!

#1 SHOW THE BOY

Let me explain this a bit. Ladies, men are visual creatures. They like seeing what they're chasing. Your favorite fluffy jammies that keep you covered from head to toe are not helping your cause in this instance. Think about it for a minute. Your coziest things are very likely not sexy. We love to pursue what we can see! I can already hear the arguments, "Doc, when we were first married, my boobs were way up here, and now they're way down here." Ladies, let me tell you something; we don't mind. We will hold them right where they belong! We will, we're nice like that. The only person who cares is you. We're big picture thinkers—we're into you, not the details! Most of the time, we are completely unaware of the details. You know that. It's true in a number of areas in our lives, and it works here too. Let me share a story to illustrate this point.

When I turned sixteen, I bought my first car for $150. It was a royal blue 1978 Pinto station wagon with no muffler. It was a chick magnet. I used to pull up to Crivitz High School and lean up next to my car like James Dean without the cigarette. I was so proud. You know why? Because it was mine. Ladies, that's the way a healthy man thinks about you. Just ask any man if he wants to see his wife when they are in bed tonight. If he's a healthy boy and a real man, you know he will. He doesn't see the stretch marks, the cellulite, and the sag you do. He sees his wife, and he's dang proud of her. That should reduce a lot of emotional stress for you ladies. If you know how this works, you can get him to do whatever you want—and you'll both be happier!

CHRISTY'S THOUGHTS

Ladies, this is so important and so SIMPLE to do, and if you value your man and your marriage, this tip will become a fun, playful habit that you will share 'till death do you part.' I guarantee that your man has some favorite 'spot' on your body, and no I'm not talking about the most obvious ones! I'm talking about that 'special spot' on your body that, when he gets a glimpse of it, drives him crazy! And ladies, it's usually a spot on your body like the nape of your neck, small of your back, or other spot that is not considered 'private.' So, use it!!! Patrick's favorite 'spot' of mine is so easy for me to just enter a room and show him purposefully—and what's the purpose? He will have ME on his mind ALL DAY LONG! When he travels this has him missing me and wanting to rush home to me as well. Ladies, it is so important to be playful with your spouse. It's healthy, and the kids don't even realize it's happening -- they just see your healthy relationship.

#2 TALK TO THE BOY

You may think you talk to him all the time. But you talk to him in a way that feeds your hormones. Right now, we are talking about his hormones. There is a way you can talk to your man to get him to do what you want him to do all day. All you have to do tomorrow morning is grab that testosterone-filled boy before he leaves for work and whisper into his ear, "Honey, tonight is going to be a good night!" What do you think your husband will be thinking about ALL DAY LONG? When he gets home, he's going to get the kids ready for bed and do the dishes. He's going to do everything he needs to do because his testosterone has been stimulated to. You have a motivated man. That's how a man works. If you don't want to do that, the sad reality is, some other woman will.

If you don't talk to him the way he needs to be talked to and you don't show him what he needs to see, some other girl will. It won't be intentional on his part. He'll be at work someday and when that pretty girl walks by and says something to him or dresses in a way that shows him a little more than he sees at home, he can't help but be stimulated. No, it's not a happy thought, but either you accept how this works, or you can be just as unhappy as the majority of marriages are today.

Has the divorce rate in the last twenty years increased or decreased? That seems to be about the timing as to when we started trying to force men to be more like women. They are what they are. When we accept that men and women were created in a specific, and different way, we'll all be able to get along much better. I know I keep hammering this point, but so do the media and our culture. Once we accept reality, we'll be able to move on from this. Until then, we'll have to continue to hammer this point over and over.

#3 DON'T FEED THE BOY

I know men like #1 and #2 but they're not going to like #3. As your husband gains too much weight, his testosterone will convert to another type of hormone, estrogens. That's why breast cancer is second to prostate cancer in men today. As their man boobs and the rest of them get larger, their hormones convert to estrogens. Fat does a very good job of producing and storing estrogens making those men become more female-like in hormone levels.

Breast cancer is second to prostate cancer in men, today.

Estrogens rising too high are a contributing factor of breast cancer. A few times after taking a man's blood work, I have had him fast for seventy-two hours and his testosterone would rise anywhere from 25-40%. Men need to cut the sugar, and men need to fast. I like to recommend a seventy-two-hour fast every three months to help with testosterone levels. Ladies, sometimes you may have to put the kibosh on him and tell him he needs to take a break for a couple of days. Remember how I told you about food and emotions? It's just as true for guys as it is for women.

#4 CAPTURE THE BOY'S MIND

My wife is a genius at this. I travel a lot. Sometimes she goes with me, but sometimes she doesn't and I'm by myself. I'm around beautiful women all the time, but it doesn't matter because Christy has learned to capture my mind. On one of my traveling tours, I found a card in my suitcase. Cool. We all love surprises. Let me read you the front of the card. "Sometimes when I look at you, I wonder how I got so lucky." Ladies swoon at this kind of stuff. You know how guys feel about it? It means nothing to a guy. But here's the part where she captured my mind: when I opened that card, right in the middle was a piece of her lingerie. All day long, I was thinking about her. That entire trip, all I was thinking about was her. She's not stupid. She knows how this works. She left that little piece of fabric there for me and captured my mind. It doesn't matter who I meet or what comes up throughout the rest of my day, she has all of my mind. I can't wait to see her again. Why? She's leveraging my testosterone and helping me stay a healthy man.

All day long, I was thinking about her. That entire trip all I was thinking about was her.

Ladies, you can help a man to be deeply focused on you and chase you the rest of your life if focus on these four things. Here's the best part—you also keep him healthy. It may sound tough or like something you may not want to do, but how much do each of these first four steps cost? Trust me, the care from our clinics is much more expensive. You don't want to have to pay us to help you get your man's testosterone back to normal. These steps cost you nothing, just a little understanding and creativity.

#5 TEST THE BOY

I often get emails and phone calls from women who have tried #1-4 to tell me it didn't work. Well, then, #5 is very important. You need to make sure he gets tested. According to his wife, over the course of the past three years, he had lost his job, gained a lot of weight, and had zero motivation. Most notably, no sexual drive. It had been two years since he'd had sex with his wife. Does that sound like a healthy boy? His wife looked at me and said, "If I wasn't a Christian woman, I would have left him already. All I have is a roommate. I don't want a roommate. I want a husband." I asked him if he had ever had his hormones tested. You can guess what his answer was. No.

But do you know what they did have him on? SIX anti-depressants. In our current way of thinking, the thought was he might have a tumor or fire of some kind. They found nothing, and since they weren't going to cut him open, it was time to use the hose. They kept adding medications. He was finally on six prescribed medications and in a horrible state! I did the obvious and measured his hormones. I sent him to the hospital where he was getting his psychiatric treatments. Take a look at his levels here:

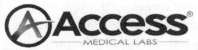

		5151 CORPORATE WAY JUPITER, FL 33458-3101 (866)720-8386	

Client: THE WELLNESS WAY	Patient: Room#: Phone:	DOB:	Age: 31 Sex:M Fasting:
GREEN BAY, WI 54313	ID#:		
Phys: FLYNN, PATRICK	Route#: 0		Page:1

ENDOCRINE EVALUATION

DHEA SULFATE	68.5	34.5 - 568.9	ng/dl
DIHYDROESTOSTERONE	12.2	11.2 - 95.5	nmo/L
TESTOSTERONE TOTAL	0.0 L	280 - 1100	ng/dl
SEX HORMONE BIND GLOBULIN	16 L	21.63 - 113.1	nmo/L
Lab Developed Testing			

Can you see his levels? No? Because they are 0! Zero. I called the hospital to see if they had made a mistake. They had him come back in and checked it four times. Four. It was consistently the same. Zero. We had figured out what triggered his fires and what he needed to rebuild his house. After three months, we ran his blood work:

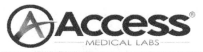

Client: THE WELLNESS WAY		Patient:				
		Room#:		DOB:	Age: 31 Sex:M	
		Phone:			Fasting:	
GREEN BAY, WI 54313		ID#:				
Phys: FLYNN, PATRICK		Route#:	0		Page:1	
ENDOCRINE EVALUATION						
TESTOSTERONE, TOTAL			717	280 - 1100	ng/dl	
SEX HORMONE BIND GLOBULIN			39	10 - 80	nmo/L	
TESTOSTERONE, FREE			13.98	1.9 - 27	ng/dl	

I had them come in to go over his labs. This time his wife's first words to me were, "Doc, turn it off !" His body had started rising back toward normal. Ladies, I have received flack for this next statement, but like I said, I speak it like it is. If your husband is not chasing you every day, it's a sign he's sick. I don't care if he's sixty or if he's twenty-five. If he's chasing you every day, he's not a pervert. He's a healthy man and you should be thanking

> **I don't care if he's sixty or if he's twenty-five, if your husband is not chasing you every day, it's a sign he's sick.**

God for that. Guys are easy to understand, easy to get back to normal, and easy to keep normal. We have a simple daily and lifelong cycle.

CHRISTY'S THOUGHTS

If only women realized that the four steps really worked and were so incredibly beneficial to men's health!! I didn't even realize that I was doing those four steps until he started pointing them out to me, or until he started using examples in his seminars. You can imagine the look on my face after I heard him bring up the 'lingerie in the card' in one of his seminars for the first time—I was probably redder than a lobster, and I guarantee my eyes were as wide as saucers!! But ladies, in all seriousness, I can handle a small bit of embarrassment if I know that it will help you with your marriage! The best advice I have for ladies to build and keep their men and marriages healthy is to do these four steps! Ladies, we need to help our men stay hormone-healthy 'till death do us part.'

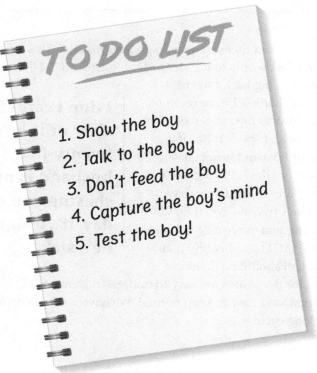

TO DO LIST

1. Show the boy
2. Talk to the boy
3. Don't feed the boy
4. Capture the boy's mind
5. Test the boy!

CHAPTER 9

WE NEED THE WHOLE PICTURE.

I wake up early in the morning to get to work on my priorities; I usually make it to the office before everyone else. I make myself a cup of good, organic coffee and sit down to read emails back in my office. One day, the first one I opened was from a man who was frustrated. His wife was exhausted, she couldn't get out of bed anymore, and she had been bleeding for over two months. The doctors couldn't find anything wrong with her.

What I read every morning frustrates me. It actually makes me sad. I sit down each morning to emails from women from all over the world who are sick. They are sick and aren't getting any help from the doctors they've entrusted with their care. Many of them have been basically told to accept what they are experiencing as their new normal. This is personal for me because my wife was once one of those women. So, early in the morning, reading all these messages, that's when I might get upset and go on a rant to tell people there's a different perspective! There's a different way of thinking than Western medicine! Can you blame me for being upset? Women's illnesses and hormone problems have skyrocketed over the years.

Doctors are not trying to not help. They are trying to do the best job they can. They just have limited resources and ways of thinking. That doesn't take away the fact that women are sick and in pain. However, their job is to keep them alive, not help them live their best life with an optimally functioning body. The current method is so incomplete that my heart breaks when they come in.

To assess a woman properly is impossible if you are trying to do it with a limited perspective.

Women have typically been to many doctors by the time they come in to see us. We are usually the last resort because we aren't part of the huge medical machine. I ask for their records and the most basic things when they come in. It is always incomplete testing that doesn't give a good picture of what is happening with them. It doesn't matter if they've been to an M.D., D.O., endocrinologist, functional medicine doctor, or other specialists. Their testing is incomplete because they simply were not taught what complete testing is, so they are unaware they aren't getting the whole picture. Even if they were, they don't know how to support the body for normal function. To assess a woman properly is impossible if you are trying to do it with a limited perspective.

Have you been at the movies watching the previews when you saw one to a movie that looked really good? Then you think, we have to see that! A few months later, you go to the movie and it's meh. You judged the movie on the preview, and you only got a small picture of what that movie was about. We have all been to a movie that had a pretty good preview, but when you saw the whole thing, it wasn't so great. We understand the preview is just a small picture. Unfortunately, that's how mainstream medicine is looking at women's hormones.

You were never taught how a woman's hormones work and we wonder why breast cancer rates are rising. We wonder why there are so many hormonal issues. If you are like most Americans, you most likely haven't been educated on how a woman's body works. That's okay, we're fixing

If you understand that each estrogen has a unique role, then you understand how damaging this can be.

that right now. How many of you have heard of the hormone estrogen? Are you ready for this? There is no such thing as a hormone called estrogen. Estrogen is a term for several different hormones that are chemically similar. They may be chemically similar, but they have different properties. With how much "high estrogen" is connected to an increased risk of breast cancer, it seems we should get to the bottom of this. Pink ribbons, mammograms, and all the research for drugs can't give you prevention. Prevention happens when you stop the condition from developing in the first place. Early detection is not the same thing. The condition has to have happened in order for you to detect it. Understanding the multiple hormones and proper testing can set your body up for health. This group of hormones influence whether you get cancer, osteoporosis, and/or heart disease. Estrogens even affect your moods—whether you are happy or depressed. Like I said, they play an important part in making up who a woman is!

Women who have been diagnosed with breast cancer will be tested to see if their type of cancer is estrogen positive. If the results say their cancer type is estrogen receptive, they will likely be put on an aromatase inhibiting drug that blocks their production of all estrogens. It's non-selective, so that means it stops the production and conversion of all the estrogens. Not just the problematic one. If you understand that each estrogen has a unique role, then you understand how damaging this can be. One of those estrogens, 2-hydroxy Estrone, is actually cancer protective. Why would you want to inhibit that one?! You wouldn't if you understood how and why it functioned that way.

All of the estrogens play an important role in making a woman who she is. Estrogen is demonized just because one type of estrogen gets out of control which can create an environment that allows breast cancer to grow and spread. Demonizing estrogen can have a detrimental effect on a body that relies on multiple estrogens for health. The other problem is that you should be thinking about how estrogen impacts your health before you have breast cancer. Why aren't we doing more to make sure women are set up for their best hormonal health? Women need to get all of their estrogens levels tested properly. That starts by knowing there is more than one.

Have you had all of those hormones tested? I ask this question of women all over the country when I speak and in my practice. I can assure you, unless they are going to a Wellness Way Clinic, they have not. Many women don't know what a proper and complete test looks like and therefore may have thought they had. Here are the markers we consider as a base in our testing at The Wellness Way:

Estrone (E1)
Estradiol (E2)
Estriol (E3)
2-OH-E1
4-OH-E1
16-OH-E1
2-Methoxy-E1
2-OH-E2
4-OH-E2
Total Estrogens

I have an idea. If one of the contributing factors to breast cancer is the level of certain estrogens, why don't we check all of the estrogen levels when women are at a young age? That makes sense.

Estrogens dictate your life, not just your breast cancer risk. It's better to prevent illness than to treat illness. But I have a question, why would we treat breast cancer if we could protect you from getting it in the first place by supporting hormonal health?

My wife had horrible health problems and painful periods. The medical community told her she would most likely not have been able to bear children. She saw lots of doctors. When I tested these hormones in my wife, I found out one of them turned her uterus into a pathological disease state. When we got that hormone back to normal levels, her uterus went back to normal. We lowered her risk for breast cancer by supporting her hormones, her health problems subsided, and her periods became normal. Testing your hormones can change your health and your life.

If your doctor has just tested your blood, there is no way you can get a true picture of all your hormones. To get a full understanding of your hormonal health, you need to utilize more than one test including:

- Blood
- Saliva
- Urine

Let me say this again so you can share with your gynecologist, your nurse practitioner, your doctor, and anyone else who just wants to draw your blood to test your hormones: It is virtually impossible to get a full picture of your hormonal health by testing blood alone.

The primary hormone they can look at through blood testing is estradiol. Conveniently, this is one they can manipulate through drugs. If you haven't had a urine test to check your hormones, you are missing important indicators. There are certain estrogens you can only see in urine. But you can't test progesterone in a urine test, so for a full hormonal picture, you will need multiple tests. I can't say this enough; a good clinical doctor will run multiple tests to get a full picture. Now think about it—did you know that there were several estrogens? Did you get multiple types of testing?

CHRISTY'S THOUGHTS

Yes, I did all three hormone tests within the same timeframe to get the proper "picture" of what was going on in my body. Everyone is different, and I cannot stress enough how important it is to get all your hormones tested and get the 'whole picture'! I have done it multiple times through the years, and my daughters will also get testing done as soon as they each begin menstruating. There is no going back to the 'common' way of doing things for us. Remember, I went to other doctors and did all their testing and got NO results and NO answers. As a result of testing thoroughly through The Wellness Way, both my life and my daughters' lives have been put on a path leading to homeostasis and away from disease. Testing is key!

Using the standard approach, women are left with incomplete information and are trusting people who are looking at an incomplete picture of the body. And we wonder why hormone conditions continue to rise. People are racing for the cure, buying the pink ribbon version of everything, attending rallies, and participating in pink 5k races–we know we have a problem, and people clearly want to help. However, imagine if this information I just shared with you was part of the conversation. We are missing the discussions that can really lead to saving lives and improved quality of health. When you understand how estrogens work and how to properly test, you can do more for prevention. It's part of a whole-body approach that understands whether you are setting your body up for health or illness.

When you start supporting a body to re-establish healthy hormones and healthy systems, your body starts responding with positive outcomes. There is more to it than just learning the names of the hormones, though. Not only do women have more hormones, but these hormones are also changing on a regular basis. Let's take a look at a chart of the typical woman's cycle.

THE FEMALE CYCLE

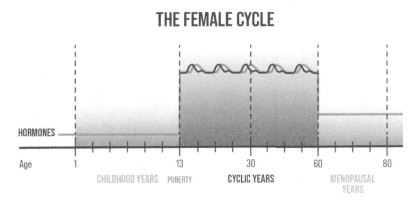

Looks quite a bit different from the graphic we looked at on men's hormones, huh?

Would you agree with me that testosterone alone causes physical and mental changes? Women have many more hormones that change throughout the month, not just throughout the day. Their cycles are very different. Their cycle and hormones affect them differently than men, both physically and mentally. Looking at the charts of the hormones, can you understand why I question how anybody can tell us that men and women are the same?

The lack of understanding of hormones is causing many of our common problems today. Even during counseling, a man is often told to be more sensitive. If a man is healthy and his testosterone levels are good, this is going to be very hard for him to do. It's denying his biology! Men are not supposed to be overly sensitive. That's not what they are. Conversely, women are supposed to be sensitive, and their hormones make their experience different than a man's. Their emotions do not mean they are crazy, it's their biology!

Understanding the different hormones and how they work can not only support a woman's health, but it can also improve her relationships.

CHRISTY'S THOUGHTS

One of the most beneficial pieces of advice I ever got was to not discuss difficult things or topics with Patrick during the day, but instead to wait. I needed to 'bridle my tongue' and talk to him at night about the issue. Ladies, we are all sensitive and emotional, but they are NOT—and that's how God made them! It's not wrong, so why not THINK DIFFERENTLY and change our approach to solving problems, instead of constantly trying to change our men??

Approach your man in the evening when his testosterone is lower and remember that it's not what you say, but HOW you say it. Speak respectfully, and he will be more likely to respond back respectfully. Your tone of voice can actually say more than you are trying to say. You could be completely right, but how you say

*something can determine whether he receives it or not. So don't try
to make him more 'sensitive'! He's a man, and a healthy man has
testosterone. If we could all (men and women) learn to control our
reactions, I think conflict resolution would not be so dreaded
or difficult.*

AMANDA'S STORY

I had been pretty healthy in my teen years. I had no
challenges with my cycles. Everything seemed just fine. The
challenges started after I decided to go off my birth control—
Depo-Provera injections.

I struggled with stage IV endometriosis and cysts
for about 10 years. I felt like I lived a double life. With
endometriosis, I looked like every other happy and healthy
person on the outside. However, at home, I spent most of my
time with a heating pad and on high doses of pain medication.
I hated to tell anyone how I was feeling. I often felt like I
was viewed as broken or just making up the symptoms.
Endometriosis is a very lonely disease. It drained me both
physically and mentally. I felt like a burden causing my family
to miss out on so many opportunities. My husband was very
supportive and stayed by my side through it all.

I tried every medication to the maximum limits – even
to the point of signing waiver forms for these higher doses –
had my uterus scraped yearly and was in a hopeless situation.
During one emergency surgery, the doctor thought the issue was
my appendix and removed it. My appendix was actually fine. I
felt like I was an experiment to the doctors I was seeing.

Everything we tried seemed to work for a month or so
before the pain returned full force. The doctors had no more
answers or treatments to try. We were out of options except for
a drastic hysterectomy, and even then, I couldn't be guaranteed
a pain-free life. All the courses of action we had taken had
damaged my body more than helped. I am still challenged by
some of the side effects of the drugs I had been given.

I found myself at my chiropractor's office, desperate for help. I was ready to try anything. When my chiropractor reached out to Dr. Patrick to consult, he looked at my tests and asked if I was a 60-year-old woman in menopause. I was a 31-year-old woman. After starting my Wellness Way journey, I was pain-free after 3 months! My chiropractor was so impacted he became a Wellness Way affiliate, so he would be able to help others.

I haven't had any medication or surgery in over two years and I'm not looking back now. In fact, I would be afraid to go back to my previous doctor—the one who "accidentally" took out my appendix. I'm afraid I would be kicked out for how strongly I feel about my health and the hope The Wellness Way has restored in my life.

It wasn't always easy, but you must do the right thing for your health. I have a supportive husband but still had a lot of criticism from those who didn't understand what I was doing and choosing. I had to choose to stay the course and do the right thing for my family, for my health.

I share my story hoping that it helps others find the help they need. I don't want anyone to have to go through a life of pain and misery that so many health challenges can cause, especially in the way of female hormones. I feel better at 33 than I did in my 20s. Thanks to The Wellness Way Approach, I have my life back, and I know they can do that for so many more people!

CHAPTER 10

WOMEN ARE COMPLICATED.
(BUT WORTH IT)

This chapter is a bit longer than the one on the man zone. Women have more hormone fluctuations and more zones. They are a bit more complicated than a man, and that's okay. That is what makes them women.

When I started researching women's hormones, one question kept jumping out at me and caused me to focus all my research on answering it. Why do women care about everything? Why do they look at everything the way they do? Let's take a day in the life of a woman. From the time a woman gets up in the morning, she is the primary person to get the kids ready for school. Have you ever seen a guy dress his kids? My wife always asks me, "How could you possibly let them leave the house dressed like that?" Sure, they might look funny, but I think, It's fine, they have clothes on. Done! We think differently.

Moms make breakfast, pack lunches, get the kids ready for school, and then drop them off. Moms pour themselves into a multitude of tasks all day, at home, the office, or both. Then, after school, they take care of the kids and have to make food again, help with homework, and after they've cared for everything all day long, they are exhausted. But she stays with this intense schedule, and every detail means so much to her, because it's what she does. She cares. About everything!

Why do women care about everything?

Now, her man left this morning, and he cared about what? Nothing! Okay, that's not to mean he doesn't care about anything, but remember, his testosterone keeps him laser-focused on one thing. He's got his "one thing" on his mind and is moving through the day. One thing at a time, one task conquered after another. He's doing great, he thinks! Triumphant, he heads home at the end of his day. What is that guy thinking when he comes home? (Insert sexy music here.)

And how does the woman respond? "Just another thing I have to do!" It's comical looking at the two perspectives, isn't it? Ladies, I hear you. This is the story you've told me for years of clinical practice and speaking tours. Guys—just understand it's a thing. It happens, and it's real. They are different from us. It's okay to be a man, but you have to understand women are very different, and it's okay to be a woman. Their hormones make them more emotional. They think differently; they care about everything. We don't. Our testosterone keeps us less emotional and only thinking about one thing at a time. We don't think about ten things at a time the way they do. That whole day means a lot to them, they poured their heart into every moment. Understand that, and you'll understand the woman.

> **It's okay to be a man, but you have to understand women are very different; and it's okay to be a woman.**

Remember back at the beginning of the book when I used the word "vagina?" I did that to illustrate a point. To understand each other, we have to be comfortable with some basics, but it's going to be tricky when the basics make many men squeamish. Women, have you ever noticed a large population of men are interested in hunting? I'm from Wisconsin, which is a big hunting state, so men and women get this analogy. A guy can go to Cabela's, buy deer urine, and spray it all over himself and the trees. He can go fishing and scrape the scales off the fish and clean them without batting an eye. He can kill a deer with either a gun or bow and field dress it right there in the woods with very few tools. But the minute a woman says she has her period, he's grossed out. Ever notice that? The irony is funny! Now this isn't every man, but I do come across it often. Guys, I know I caught your attention with the "v word," but I promise I won't use the word vagina anymore. Don't worry, we'll still communicate effectively.

Let's go back to my analogy and use the example of a house. For the rest of the section, we'll look at the female cycle from a man's point of view. If a female is a house in this analogy, we'll call the word I promised not to say, "the man cave." Not because the man owns it! Rather, of all the places in the house a man may enjoy, the man cave is his favorite spot. In this house, the man cave changes on a regular basis. Why? There are physical and mental changes going on. All the time. This is what a cycle looks like for a woman through the course of a month:

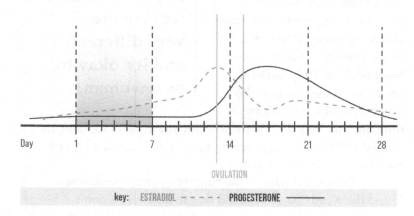

A woman's cycle can range from twenty-six to thirty-two days. It can be twenty-seven one time and twenty-nine another and still considered normal. It doesn't have to be the exact same every time. The average cycle for women is about twenty-eight days.

Let's look at the hormone patterns. These patterns should change four times a month. When I got married, my wife looked at me after our pastor said our vows and said, "I do." Guys, it's different for us. The pastor should have asked us to say, "I do" four times. When you say "I do" to a woman, you are really marrying four different women, depending on which week of her cycle she is in. I'm going to show you how this works, and it's not as weird as it may sound. Have you ever noticed sometimes life with your wife can be really awesome, and then the following week, all you are thinking is who did I marry?! You think she's a totally different person. Guys, you know it's true, but you also have to know that sometimes the personality shift is just fine and even okay. Men (and women) don't understand so they think there's something wrong with them when this happens. And when the man tells her she has to be like him, it only makes it worse. Today's sexual revolution is telling us that women can be as sexually driven as men. They can work to the same level as men, they can exercise as hard as they want, as consistently as they want. Please don't buy into that—they may be able to pull it off for a time, but they shouldn't. If they are as driven as men, they are sick. Let me say it again. If a woman has a sex drive like a man, she is likely on the road to being sick and will probably develop cancer someday if those hormone levels don't fall back into the normal female ranges. Let me explain the woman zones.

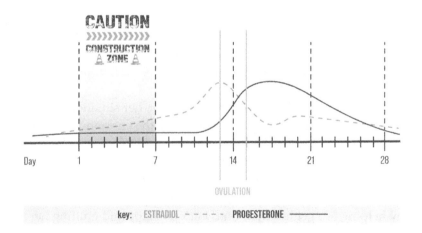

ZONE 1 : THE CONSTRUCTION ZONE

This is when the cycle starts. The bleeding period can go anywhere between four to seven days. This is when the man cave is under construction. Her hormones change, and the first two weeks of her cycle are dominated by estrogens. The construction zone is a very important time during a woman's cycle and is an integral part of keeping hormones healthy. The body is under a certain amount of stress because it is under

construction. It takes work and resources for the body to
properly undergo this process.

I want to see normal hormones and keep it that way to prevent fires.

Women turn to me
when their hormones show
their bodies are in distress.
That's how I ended up with a
baseball-sized blood clot on my
desk. Okay, I'm a doctor and
all, and totally comfortable with
anatomy but this was a doozy
even for me! A patient I was
working with who had endometriosis came into my office just
after her period started and placed a plastic baggie with a giant
blood clot in it on my desk.

Yes, a plastic baggie.

Yes, a baseball-sized blood clot. I can still picture it. She
asked me, "What do you think about that?"

I paused, then slowly said, "Well...I don't think it
belongs on my desk!"

We laughed, but despite the humor, her situation
wasn't funny. You see, I didn't need to see the enormous clot to
understand the pain she was experiencing. I have supported,
and continue to support, many women who are facing a similar
experience. She knew I dealt with these types of issues all the
time, so she trusted me enough to bring in her clot. I responded
by helping her get her hormones back in shape and guiding her
back to homeostasis.

There is a lot you can learn when women trust you and
share their experiences with you.

When we test, we are working to keep tabs on those
levels and prevent, or help our patients recover from the
devastation of disease, or fire that could result. When someone's
body is trying to adapt to stress, their body could have trouble
making or converting hormones. Simply stated, those hormones
are getting thrown off. However, until you develop a serious

condition, and your house is actually on fire, the fire department won't show up.

Estrogens are produced by the ovaries. That's important, because later in the month this hormone production will change. What do estrogens do for women? They make them energetic, outgoing, social, and enthusiastic, and they also alter their metabolism, causing them to eat about 15% less than men. Estrogens also increases their serotonin—the happy hormone.

Men, pay attention. When the man cave is under construction, more oxytocin is released, and her love hormone goes up. Estrogens tell a woman's brain to connect. They don't say "go get it" like your testosterone. Guys please learn this—it will be life-changing. Every guy knows when a woman starts her cycle, the man cave is unavailable, and he won't be able to visit it anytime soon. He disconnects because he doesn't see the purpose. Again ladies, this is not because we are jerks, just testosterone driven, focus-on-the-moment guys. But guys, day one of a cycle is where you can make your wife very sick. Her love hormone has increased and because our sex drive can't be fulfilled, we think we are respecting her by not "pestering." Fair thought. However, she needs you and she needs you in a very specific way, maybe just not the way you think. When you separate from her, her love hormone and estrogens drop.

We have to understand, guys, it's okay for you to have a sex drive, but this is how her body works so you have to put her needs above yours during this zone. Your sex drive will still be there when it's over, and you want her to be healthy. When her period comes, it's your job to work at connecting with her. This is key to keeping her healthy. Ask her how her day was and what's happening in her life. If she just says everything is fine, then dig a little deeper. Do things that she enjoys doing. I take my wife dancing, but that might not be what your wife likes. Do what she likes. Watch the romantic comedy, take a walk with her, fix her favorite dinner, or whatever it is she likes. The most important thing is that she feels connected and loved.

Here's an interesting tidbit about working out. Ladies, if you exercise intensely during The Construction Zone, you run the risk of affecting your hormones and pushing your body to be stressed. Your body then thinks it has to produce more hormones. There is one tissue that does a really good job of making hormones— adipose tissue, or fat. Yes, the very thing you are trying to avoid! If you push your body during the wrong times of the month during the wrong zones you can exercise all you want, and you'll gain more fat. Another reason why understanding your physiology is important.

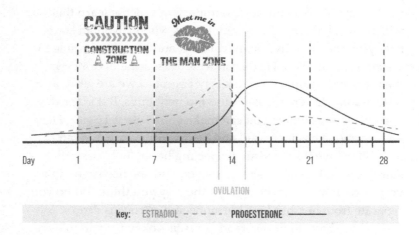

ZONE 2 : THE MAN ZONE

When the period stops, and her hormones have come up properly, she enters the Zone men are eagerly waiting for. She becomes similar to a man in her sex drive. A woman in her Zone 1 doesn't have much of a sex drive, but as everything increases, so does that libido. It's okay and very normal for her sex drive to match her man's at this time.

Let's look at those estrogens and how to support them again. This is the week to exercise. In the Man Zone, it's very important for ladies to exercise. Their bodies can handle it. They also handle stress better, it may even seem like nothing bothers them. Women also burn sugar better in this zone. Have you noticed there are times when you can eat anything and not gain a pound and other times you eat an organic salad and gain five? It's probably the same week your husband gives up soda and loses twenty pounds. We know—it's annoying.

Men, these first weeks help feed her body the right way. We're talking about serotonin, fatty acid, estrogen-based foods. Let's picture a stressed-out woman. Her day was terrible, her husband was frustrating, work was horrible, her kids are driving her nuts and she's craving an organic salad. Does that sound right to you? No! I've never heard a woman say that. When you are stressed, what does your body crave? Chocolate! Do you know why? Chocolate has the highest serotonin content of any food on the planet. Your body knew exactly what it was doing when it sent that craving message.

When I started understanding this, I studied chocolate like crazy. Hershey still sells more chocolate than anyone else in the world. Valentine's Day, four billion Hershey's kisses are sold! When I'm talking about the health benefits of chocolate, I'm not talking about Hershey or any other highly-processed chocolate–those are filled with sugar and chemicals. I'm talking about healthy, real food. Raw cacao is actually a superfood with a ton of benefits. There's a very big difference between it and what you can find on display by the register at the grocery store. Don't reach for the bad stuff. That isn't the message your body is sending!

> **It's very difficult for a woman. Their bodies change four times in a month!**

Men, here's a valuable "insider secret." There are many different forms of chocolate. There are cacao beans, nibs, powder, paste, but let me tell you about a little gem called cacao butter. You should feel my hands. They're pretty nice for a guy's hands. Let me tell you why. When my wife has her period, I'll take some cacao butter and coconut oil and I'll start rubbing her down and massaging her with it. Why? Because I'm a nice guy? Well, I'm nice, but giving massages isn't exactly my favorite pastime. But I understand how cacao benefits women, so I'm trying to make sure that while she's under the Construction Zone, I'm going to do everything I can to get her into the Man Zone and keep her there for as long as is healthy. I rub her down and feed her body by rubbing healthy oils and fats on her skin. My hands are so nice because I understand it's my role as her husband to help her through Zone 1 so we can get to Zone 2 and make sure Zone 2 is as good as it can be. Guys, we do have it easy. We keep our testosterone good and things are really simple for us. It's very difficult for a woman. Their bodies change four times in a month. FOUR! I keep saying it, and I will until every man and woman realizes this is normal, not crazy.

By looking at things from a different perspective, we can help you figure out what specifically each woman needs. We want husbands to understand this as well because as their wife's body is going through that transition, he should help her with this. You are a team, and, up until now, I suspect that no one has ever taught you how to support each other's hormone health.

I had a woman come in who was dealing with what I'll call "man cave dryness" (you know what I mean). She sent me an email after I figured out what her body needed, and she started taking steps to correct her situation. Here's the email:

Dr. Patrick, I wanted to update you and thank you for the advice you gave my husband and me at our last appointment. When you told me the benefits of coconut oil and cacao butter and how they affects the vaginal tissue, I thought you were a little bit crazy. But you've given me good advice so far, so we decided to try it. After applying it vaginally for a couple of days, we started to notice that the soreness started to go down, so we decided to try it out. After a couple of weeks, I'm happy to tell you that I'm starting to enjoy sex again and my husband is very pleased. Not just because we've had more sex in the last couple of weeks than we've had in the last year, but my husband

and I have been able to get into positions that I have not been in for over thirty years. He thanks you! Your advice has helped me physically, mentally and brought me closer to my husband.

She's eighty-three years young. Can you believe it? It goes to show your body is meant to function optimally no matter what your age is!

Alright guys, here's the first of your two To Do Lists:

#1 FEED THE GIRL

I'm going to help you guys read a woman's mind. Not all of it; testosterone or no, we aren't equipped for that! Here is the most important thing that you can help with on a regular basis, "Feed me chocolate and tell me I'm pretty." She needs the chocolate and loves the reassurance. Remember she doesn't have testosterone telling her how awesome she is. It's your job to tell her. It was part of the marriage agreement when you said, "I do" to your four wives.

Ladies, if you fast, especially during from the right foods at the wrong times, you'll be very sick. Feed the hormones. For a guy you need to create a bit of stress to support their hormones; this is just one more way we are very different. That's why women can eat hardly anything and still be overweight. Men, in the first two weeks of her cycle, help them with this. Provide the things they need to feed their hormones. They need it—the results will prove it to you. People are blown away because after doing the most simple and basic things, their bodies begin changing like crazy. During the first two weeks of her cycle, a woman needs to be eating foods high in fatty acids.

> **Remember, she doesn't have testosterone telling her how awesome she is.**

Here's your shopping list:

- Chocolate-the good kind!
- Chia seeds
- Pumpkin seeds
- Sunflower seeds
- Coconut products
- Walnuts
- Pecans and most other nuts
- Olive oil
- Hemp
- Dates
- Avocados
- Cherries
- Grapes (organic wine is okay)
- Maca

#2 TALK TO THE GIRL

Now that the ladies have read the first part of the book the guys are loving life. Their ladies are taking care of them and understand how their guys work. If guys are confused, they may walk up to their ladies in the morning (because they think their lady is just like them) and

> We see the kind of "guy phrases" in movies and while guys think it's great, girls think it's stupid.

say "Honey, tonight is going to be a good night!" Guess what is going to happen. Your wife is NOT going to come home that night. Why? That doesn't connect with a woman. Don't speak to a woman that way—they need more finesse! We see the idea of "guy phrases" in movies, and while guys think it's great, girls think it's stupid. They know that's not how it works. That doesn't appeal to a woman. Women need connecting words.

There are three words that appeal to a woman. Guys may think it doesn't matter, because she knows it already, but ask my wife. I tell her this all the time. I text her this phrase early in the morning and I'll text it to her in the afternoon. What are the three most important words you can say to a woman? Hint: it's not "I love you."

It's "I choose you." That is one of the most connecting things you can say to a woman. When you disconnect from her, she feels left alone. When she feels disconnected, she'll create things in her head. When you disconnect with her, she thinks you're connecting with someone else. She really does. And she'll play it over in her head and she'll create scenarios and the weirdest things you will ever hear in your life. Most of us have been through it.

Several years ago, as I was getting ready to speak to a group, my wife sent me a text message. I thought that was odd, she doesn't send me a text when she knows I'm getting ready to go on stage. But this was special. My thirteen-year-old daughter was at her first dance at her Christian school. All the girls were standing, swaying back and forth in their pretty dresses. What do you think they were all thinking? Come, choose me! To women this is sweet and precious. Then, two minutes later, she sent me a picture with this cute thirteen-year-old blonde boy dancing with my daughter. It meant so much to my wife, because every woman, my wife included, knows how important it is to feel chosen. Guys are different so all I could think is, "where's my gun?" He may be sweet, but I turned into protective Papa Bear in a heartbeat! I know what those pubescent boys are like and what his hormones are saying...back to the ladies. Every woman loves to be pursued, to know that she is the focus of her man's affection. It's in their biology. Guys, when you don't chase them, they start to feel disconnected from you.

I've made an observation. Watch out for your friends, ladies. When one of them goes through a divorce or another stressful time, no matter the age, they get very sick quickly. They just do. When a woman feels disconnected and goes through a bad relationship, her hormones drop. Ladies, here's a tip. When your friend is going through a lot of stress, sometimes women can pick up the slack where men are not. That's sad, isn't it ? Your friends can help you out just by being a connecting friend. Guys, you can't help each other out that way. Our testosterone won't be driven up by connecting to another man. We're not wired that way.

CHRISTY'S THOUGHTS

To be chosen...over and over again...it's the most amazing feeling, isn't it? You know what we do every day to keep our relationship playful and alive? Patrick and I have our own 'code' that we send each other via emojis! Between emojis and GIFs, we stay connected all throughout each day, even we are too busy to talk. Be creative and playful in your relationships and you will be pleasantly surprised by how close you become. And ladies, you can be an ear to listen to your girlfriends when they are going through stress. Just listen and connect, and you will help reduce her stress.

One piece of advice from what I have observed though -- ladies, if you are struggling in your marriage, guard your heart and do not talk and connect with other men. Ladies should connect with ladies, and guys should talk to guys when it comes to marriage issues and counseling. Just as my husband mentioned in the chapter on testosterone-guys, if you stress your woman out and you don't go out of your way to try to connect with her and she starts talking and connecting with another man, you may be heading in a dangerous direction of destruction in your marriage. Three little words: I Choose You. Connect, connect, connect, this can mean the difference between a healthy, vibrant marriage and one that is stagnant and dysfunctional. Love is a verb -- you need to choose to actively love your spouse in the way that they receive it best!

#3 TOUCH THE GIRL

I have gotten thousands of emails on this one. Guys, the light switches for the man cave are not inside the man cave. Simple as that.

A woman's hormones (including her emotional connection and even physical reception to affection) fluctuate four times a month. Finding the light switches can be an adventure. It's like looking for Waldo in a different place every week. You know this, because you think, I've got this. It was a good night. I touched her there and she loved it. Next week you go to touch her there and she's all: "DON'T touch me!" She's not crazy. Her body changed. One area that was sensitive and felt good one week doesn't feel as good the following week. Guys, when they touch us, it feels good all the time. Right? Just make it a game and try to find those light switches. I've had emails that have said it's changed people's marriages, just knowing they each like to be touched differently. She's not him and when he gets that, they're both good.

> **It's like looking for Waldo in a different place every week.**

ZONE 3 : THE WOMAN ZONE

In the middle of her cycle, you have a totally different woman in your house because her hormones are totally different.

TO DO LIST

1. Feed the girl
2. Talk to the girl
3. "I Choose YOU!"
4. Touch the girl

127

Ladies, hear this clearly: you are normal. You ladies will come to me because your emotions change, and you feel bad. Please—you don't need to feel bad! Just like your husband has no control over his morning testosterone, you have no control over your hormones and emotions changing. None. That should give you ladies a lot of mental peace. You are not supposed to have your emotions flat lined. It's okay for you to go up and down. There's nothing wrong with that. Look what happens in Zone 3:

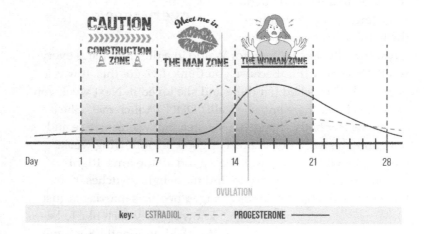

Be very careful guys, you don't know who you are coming home to during this zone. I mean this sincerely; she may bite you. Ok, not literally! Just know she's normal. Don't make her feel bad because she's emotional and her body is more sensitive to these changes.

With the switch of the hormones, her adrenals take over instead of the ovaries like we talked about during the first half of the cycle. Adrenals are the "stress glands." If your body hasn't been adjusted, has chemical stress, physical stress, and you are emotionally stressed out, this is the week that could make you very sick. If you exercise too hard during this week, it may affect your hormones and cause even more stress. If you start to stress out, your body will go into the stress response; stress affects your progesterone. Your body needs to relax, and progesterone is a calming hormone. The main job of progesterone is to balance what estrogens do so that they don't become a problem.

Let's look at a seventy-year-old patient. This woman had gone to her medical doctor, and by the time she had gotten to us, she was already taking two anti-depressants. She wanted to get off them because she felt she was getting worse. Her son, who is in his fifties, brought her into our office. We had helped guide him and he saw how it had changed his life; he knew we could help her. She had gone through all the tests and exams her general practitioner would have her do and since they hadn't found anything, they put her on a psychiatric drug. They did what they knew, but I asked her if they had ever tested her hormones. The answer was no.

> **If you start to stress out, your body will go into the stress response; stress reduces your progesterone.**

I started with the proper hormone testing. Come to find out, her progesterone levels were at zero. She sat with me and her son and as we were going over her tests and she started crying. She said three words, "I'm not crazy." Don't confuse hormonal problems with psychiatric problems. There could be something more going on. I wonder how many women

ST. VINCENT HOSPITAL   835 S. VANBUREN ST., GREEN BAY, WI   54301   CLINICAL LABORATORY REPORT

PATIENT: LOC:
M.R. #:   AGE: SEX: F
ACCT. #:   DOB:
                              DOCTOR: FLYNN, PATRICK MICHAEL   PAGE: 1

   W20576 COLL: 01/29/2014 11:51 REC: 01/29/2014 11:56 PHYS: FLYNN, PATRICK MICHAEL

   SEND OUT TEST
     ASSAY NAME   TJ UPTAKE
     TESTING LAB: QUEST / NICHOLS INTITUTE LAB
     TEST RESULTS: SEE QUEST DIAGNOSTICS REPORT
     REF. RANGE: SCANNED IN EPIC

   W20574 COLL: 01/29/2014 11:52 REC: 01/29/2014 11:57 PHYS: FLYNN, PATRICK MICHAEL
     CORTISOL

PROGESTERONE	0.00	ng/mL

   PROGESTERONE   0.00   ng/mL
                        Female Progesterone Reference Range:
                        Ovulatory Cycle:
                           Follicular: 0.15 - 1.40 ng/mL
                           Luteal: 3.34 - 25.56 ng/mL

will spend their whole lives thinking they are crazy like this poor woman did. I'm frustrated and I'm not even one of these women! That woman was seventy, let's look at the other end of the spectrum.

> **Don't confuse hormonal problems with psychiatric problems.**

Before I tell this story, I want to assure you I'm sharing this information with your best interest at heart. I have four daughters, and I have to deal with this personally. Be very careful letting your young daughters play sports. Not that they are incapable, but if they get heavily involved and are consistently doing high levels of physically intense activity, they can affect their hormone levels. Knowing what we know about female hormones, you can see the problems this can mean for them. Boys are very different—a good way of building testosterone is moving and exercise. Protect your young girls from the kind of stressors that will affect their hormones. Teach them how to work within their cycle.

One patient I had was nineteen-year-old woman, a runner, and a Division 1 scholarship winner for track and field. Do you know what often happens to women runners' cycles? It's called amenorrhea, the absence of a period. It's common, but that doesn't mean it is normal. The school told her if she didn't

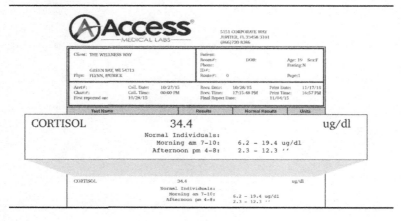

run, they'd pull her scholarship. So, as a result, she's physically stressed, mentally stressed, and affected her cycle. Why? When you rev the engine really high and don't know how to fuel it, you're going to affect your normal physiology. We tested her stress hormone. It was so high, it was double the chart's highest value. Yes, you can test stress hormone. It's called cortisol.

Remember, specific hormones are typically higher in the morning, to help you get through the day, and become lower at night, only to rebuild again. If the levels of certain hormones are very high all the time, the body may be under chronic stress. If the levels go very low and decline too quickly or too far, you experience fatigue. What's the second most common diagnosis given to women today? Chronic Fatigue Syndrome. Let me guess how many of you have had your cortisol tested. Your stress hormones can actually tell your doctor where your body is functioning, high stress or fatigue. The whole key is this, we don't test for fires, we test for function. It's very important to get your stress hormones tested, especially if you are a woman. How we take care of you differs as those hormones fluctuate.

CHRISTY'S THOUGHTS

I agree that sports can be detrimental to a young woman's health. That's why testing and knowledge about hormones and how to become and stay healthy is so crucial. But I would add that it doesn't have to be sports -- college itself can be stressful. The stress that I experienced in college was depleting my hormones to the point that I felt like every organ in my body was shutting down. From having migraines every day for an entire semester, to not being able to eat without cramping or becoming ill, to having periodic chest pains, anxiety attacks, and female issues. Stress was successfully shutting my body down. I chose to lessen my stress load by changing my major.

It was bittersweet, but my health was more important to me than getting a certain degree. What I didn't realize at that time was that God had bigger plans for me than the small plans I had for myself. Don't put unreasonable expectations on yourself or your children, especially if they are female. I was the one who put the high expectations on myself, and I suffered as a result. I wish I had known more about hormone health back then. You can't change the past, but you can affect the future. I will definitely be advocating for my children so that we can enjoy grandchildren someday!!

Some women tell me they are more of a night person than a morning person. That may seem harmless enough, but it's actually an indicator that they are functioning on an atypical hormonal pattern. Hormones, and correspondingly energy, are supposed to be highest in the morning. If you have a hard time getting through the morning, and at night when you are not supposed to have much hormone, you feel you can take on the world, your rhythms are likely off. You are supposed to rest at night. Most people we see have too much hormone at night and not enough during the day. That's why we ask patients if they are night people or morning people—it's a great clue for us. If their hormones aren't reaching the right levels at the proper times, that's why they struggle to get their bodies out of bed. At night when you don't need as much, every little bit feels like enough to keep powering through. Now this is a tough one, because most women say they feel fine. They report having a hard time getting out of bed and better able to get a lot done at night. They don't want us to mess up that energy! I understand that, but health needs to come first.

ZONE 4 : THE BONUS ZONE

If all of these changes happen as the month goes on, and she isn't properly supported, this last zone can be unknown.

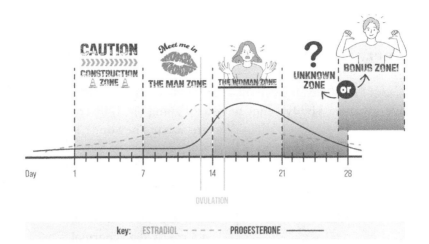

Men, you don't know who you are walking into the house to meet that day. But if you take the advice I give you, make sure she is tested properly, and help that woman through her cycle, you'll enter the Bonus Zone! This is when libido soars and she becomes similar to you in libido and energy again. If her hormones have not been properly supported up until this point, then it's back to the Woman Zone. How's that for motivation to help your wife out?

Ladies, let me give you a little mental peace. Honestly, you should only have a sex drive about two weeks of the month. Let me say that again. Physiologically you should only have a sex drive two weeks of the month. If you have a sex drive all month long, I am concerned you have abnormal hormones which can lead to you having illness down the road. You are likely either sick or on your way to becoming sick and better get checked out. Your husband will be happy, but your hormones are likely in abnormal ranges and you may be facing some health conditions.

This final week is the week that will let you know how you did the first three weeks of the month. We either have another Man Zone or another Woman Zone. I think we can all agree which we'd prefer— healthy hormones!

Okay guys, here's your second To Do List:

#1 HELP THE GIRL

I don't just believe this, I know this. It's very difficult to have a woman's body—they have a lot going on. They change every week. They don't always understand this, so they think there is something wrong with them. Ladies, there's nothing wrong, it's what your body does. Help her to know she is not crazy, she is normal.

> **Ladies, there's nothing wrong. It's what your body does.**

Help her deal with stress and life. Help her make wise food choices. Help her.

CHRISTY'S THOUGHTS

I know that there is a very large feminist movement of women who want to 'do everything a man can,' but I disagree! Women have become so sick as a result of this faulty thinking. Our bodies were not meant to take on that much stress. And there is nothing wrong with that. It doesn't mean that women are not capable or can't have certain positions or roles in companies. Some of our top VPs and earners (doctors and practitioners) in our companies are women. But my husband and I understand how much stress they can handle, and he is committed to teaching all of our staff and their spouses about setting priorities and making sure to use time management effectively in accomplishing their priorities. We women can do one thing a man CAN'T, and that is bear children. God created us to be able to have children, and, in my opinion, it is an amazing gift that should not be taken lightly. There are so many women, just like me, who have been lied to and told they cannot have children. I disagree!

A few years ago, I lost my mother. Patrick, knowing that my family is on my priority list, was able to help me to spend the time I needed with my family. Patrick was able to take on more responsibility that I normally took care of at home so that I could be with my dad and siblings as we dealt with funeral arrangements and spent much needed time with each other. That's what Patrick means by 'helping your wife.' If you can successfully fulfill your priorities with effective time management, you can insert yourself into your spouse's schedule to help them accomplish what they need to get done on their priority list. Patrick does this all the time! I don't expect it though. We talk over our weekly schedules on Sundays, and then, if he is able, he can insert his ability to help me. Now ladies, I feel like I do need to mention that if your husband is offering to help you, and it's something that doesn't need specific instruction, please let him do it HIS way. Like doing the dishes or cleaning or getting the kids ready for school or bed—if he is offering to do it, girl, you need to step aside and let him do it!! Likewise, if he is offering to do something that would actually cause you more stress, just simply thank him and politely decline, but offer something else that he can do to help you. Ladies, if he wants to help you, you need to let him help you, and, although he may think he is Superman, he cannot read your mind.

#2 DON'T STRESS THE GIRL

You can be the greatest thing to help her be healthy or the biggest factor in making her sick. Please don't be that kind of guy. It's really sad, but guys don't understand this, and neither do women. Let me give you an example of a situation I had in San Francisco. I was speaking and a woman who considered herself a feminist came up to me and said, "Doctor, I disagree. I can handle just as much stress as a man." I asked her why she was there. She said, "Because I'm sick." I told her, "Take a seat, I think you may be surprised at what you learn today." I wasn't being disrespectful, but I understand the body doesn't function based on your beliefs.

You don't have to believe me—the research has been done, and you can find it in books as well as online. Mental stress will affect your hormones. Physical stress will affect your hormones. Chemicals will affect your hormones. Guys are lucky in that stress does not affect our hormones as much as it does a woman's. The guy can have a horrible day. Work was challenging, the kids' behavior sucked, and still, he gets home at night and what does he want? SEX. If a lady has stress, and guys, you know there's very little chance of visiting the man cave that night. Those panties are super-glued in place. Right?

Men, it's your job to reduce the stress of a woman.

Why? It changes their body when they stress out. Ladies, you may not want to hear this, but take comfort in it: you are not designed to handle stress like a man, your biology will never allow it to happen. Men, it's your job to reduce the stress of a woman. This alone should relieve stress for women.

#3 PROTECT THE GIRL

I got home one day, and I could tell right away that my wife and daughter were having a challenging time. Christy told me, "Go talk to your daughter!"

So, I took Faith to our favorite organic tea spot, and after a little chatting she starts, "Daddy..."

I interrupted her, "Whoa, whoa, whoa, before you say anything, remember this, that's my wife. I will protect my wife from anybody, including you. So, when you go home, you're going to go and apologize to your mother. Remember, if you make her stressed out, you can make her sick. You are eventually going to grow up and leave her, I'm not."

After a while, we went home, and they talked. I still to this day don't even know what the problem was. The next morning when I went to wake Faith, she said, "Daddy, before you go, I just want to say I'm sorry for making Mom mad last night."

I told her, "Don't worry, God forgives, just move on." She went on to say, "Daddy, I've been thinking about it a lot. I know why I drive Mom so crazy."

"Really, you do?"

"Yeah, I'm just like you!" I laughed like crazy. Oh my goodness—where did she come up with that?! Christy would tell you she's the image of me in every way. It's worth noting: Bond to your wife. She needs you two to stay connected. Protect her, even from her own kids and yourself. When guys get stressed or face a challenge, they won't stop thinking about it until there is a solution. They may feel disconnected from everyone around them. You've heard the expression home, but not home? A guy can be physically present and a million miles away at the same time. Your wife needs the connection.

#4 SCHEDULE WITH THE GIRL

The greatest thing a guy could say to his wife in the morning would be, "Honey, would you like to go on a date with me?" Oh guys, if you could only see the room full of smiling ladies I see when I say this in one of my seminars. Guys, when you first met that woman, you did everything. Your testosterone was driven, you created pictures in your mind, you chased her, you dated her, and you scheduled things with her. She's still the same way, but most guys have stopped doing those things. Her biology will always desire to connect with you. One of the best things guys can do is to continue to date their wives. If you do this, and you plan it, she'll create the picture in her mind of all the wonderful things that make you to be the most amazing man in her world. I still date my wife! I plan it all, including the dance classes that I once signed us up for. I told her in advance, and she was so excited before our date and beaming after our date. My wife likes dancing, you will have to think about what your wife likes. It doesn't have to be fancy if you show her that you see her and understand her. Guys, how much does that cost you? A little effort perhaps, but it pays off huge. Plan it. YOU plan it, guys. When you were first

> **One of the best things guys can do is to continue to date their wives.**

chasing her and pursuing her, you planned everything. That connects with her. Then when you married her, it became, "What do you want to do?" Don't take that easy way out.

Take her somewhere peaceful to sit and just ask her, "Honey, how was your day?" That gives a woman the opportunity to talk for the next three-and-a-half hours and you don't have to do anything. No joke! But when she talks, she's connecting. What does that do to her hormones? It makes her healthy. Think about that. It's very simple.

Now I hear, "Doc, we do all of these things, and my wife still doesn't respond."

#5 TEST THE GIRL

Today, women deal with hormonal problems more than ever in history, and they are as sick as can be, and aren't getting the answers they need. It's why we have more fertility problems and more cancers. This health restoration concept we started years ago has become a brand with international awareness for this reason. It's a different thought process that's easy to apply with a doctor open to a different perspective. When we apply this different perspective to patients, we get different results -- results completely different from what the mainstream medicine approach can achieve. Right now, based on medical statistics, heart disease rates are going up and cancer rates are going up. If you don't change your thinking, you're likely going to end up as one of those statistics. My wife could have been one

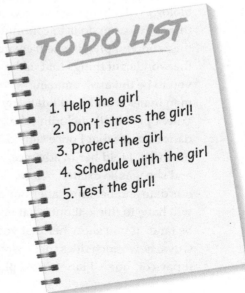

TO DO LIST

1. Help the girl
2. Don't stress the girl!
3. Protect the girl
4. Schedule with the girl
5. Test the girl!

of those statistics. This is very real. Remember, don't accept common for normal.

JOY'S STORY

I had been a healthy young woman until I went off the Depo-Provera injections which I was using as birth control. The years leading up to our Wellness Way journey had been filled with tons of attempts to find natural remedies to balance my hormones and tons of frustration and disappointment with each one. I was almost 30 years old. My husband and I had been married for 10 years. By this time, we had a miscarriage and lost twins. I was heartbroken and losing hope of having children.

To top things off, I had just had my adrenal function tested and was told I'd be on medication for the rest of my life.

From the moment we walked into The Wellness Way and our first appointment with Dr. Patrick, things were different. He was so upbeat and positive, even after we shared the adrenal test results with him. This was the first time I'd ever seen a doctor upbeat or positive after looking at my situation. To be honest, this was what gave me hope to continue on. In fact, during our first appointment he said, "Give me six months, and you'll be pregnant!" How could I not have hope?

Well, sure enough, we had our first baby girl in 2009! We were so excited when we conceived our miracle. You can only imagine our surprise and amazement when three months later we conceived our second baby girl! Fifteen months after our second daughter was born, we conceived our son.

Not only was Dr. Patrick invaluable in helping us start our family, but with two babies so close together, and a third shortly after you can only imagine all the hormone fluctuations. He was an amazing help through breastfeeding, post-partum care and nearly back-to-back pregnancies. And those adrenals? No problem.

One thing I can say about Dr. Patrick, when he gets your hormones where they need to be, they work just fine!

CHAPTER 11

NO CONTROL WITH BIRTH CONTROL.

This happens every day, imagine the day in the life of an average couple. Mackenzie looks up briefly as her husband, Adam, gets home and returns to scrubbing the counter. As he walks in, Adam senses something isn't right. He asks, "Mackenzie, is something wrong?" She looks up exasperated. He doesn't know what to do, so he moves to hug her. As soon as he touches her, Mackenzie gets so frustrated she wants to scream, but she doesn't know why, so instead she starts to cry. She shakes uncontrollably as she cries and pushes him away. Neither of them connects it right away to the birth control pill Mackenzie recently started taking. It sounds dramatic, but I have heard stories like this many times before.

Many women don't connect their hormone problems and other ailments to this common endocrine disruptor. Over half of women between the ages of fifteen and forty-four have used the birth control pill at some point in their lives for contraceptive purposes. Very few of those women have taken out their magnifying glass to look at the FDA approved product insert that comes with that monthly prescription. If they did, they would see a long list of side effects.

Some of the Potential Risks, Side Effects and Adverse Reactions Listed in the Insert:

- Risk of developing blood clots
- Heart attacks and strokes
- Gallbladder disease
- Liver tumors
- Cancer of the reproductive organs and breasts
- Irregular vaginal bleeding
- Changes in vision
- Melasma
- Change in appetite
- Nausea
- Headache
- Nervousness
- Mental Depression

- Dizziness
- Loss of scalp hair
- Rash
- Vaginal infections
- Allergic reactions
- Gastrointestinal Symptoms
- Weight gain
- Vaginal candidiasis
- Pre-menstrual syndrome
- Acne
- Changes in libido

The list should tell you something -- don't mess with the female body! When you interfere with the delicate balance of hormones, you can cause such devastation to her body. The minute you disrupt one hormone in a female's body, it can set off a cascade of bad side effects.

Birth control itself is an endocrine disruptor. It disrupts your hormones which will disrupt all of the systems like the gears in the Swiss watch. This common pill will alter your whole endocrine system, it's what it is designed to do, which determines much of your life.

When you start taking birth control pills you are giving your body synthetic hormones, so your body stops making them itself.

When you start taking birth control pills you are giving your body endocrine disruptors that will affect the production of your natural hormones This means your hormones are being manipulated synthetically, and so is your body's production of hormones. This prohibits your body's natural and proper function. That disruption sets your body up for problems now and even more problems down the road.

When you were a young lady and started your cycle, your genes did not change, your habits did not change—your hormones changed. It changed your whole body, including your thinking, and now you're going to take a disruptor. Knowing what you now know about female hormones, do you really think it's going to be okay?

Society has come to think hormonal birth control is harmless. Sometimes we are even told it's beneficial! I'm telling you now, it's neither harmless nor beneficial. These prescriptions cause a host of complications like infertility, cancer, hormone imbalance, and low libido. The convenience they offer is surely not worth the damage. No, it's not a popular stance to take, but it's an important one. The conditions that are terrible consequences of these drugs are on the rise, and often the damage is irreversible. I will continue to share the truth until we see all these conditions disappear. We need to stop sacrificing the health of women for convenience.

The couple from our scenario likely decided that Mackenzie would go on birth control to prevent pregnancy until they were ready to have kids. This is a decision many couples make. The pill was the option they chose so they could have sex without worrying about pregnancy. Ironically, they have started a new cascade of worries. How intimate can a couple get if her hormones are out of balance? Quite frankly, intimacy is typically the last thing a woman is interested in if they have gained weight, have headaches, depression, vaginal infections, or any other side effects.

When they are ready to have that baby, will her body be ready? Her hormones have been disrupted for so long, we don't know what they will be like. They might find her hormones don't just come back after she stops taking the pill. When Mackenzie and Adam want to have kids, they may run into fertility problems. Then we will have to work on rebuilding Mackenzie's hormones. It could take lots of heartbreak and unnecessary spending to rebuild hormones because they were destroyed by this endocrine disruptor. Not everyone is lucky enough to restore them.

Some women do everything in their routine naturally, but then they take birth control because their husband wants them to. I wonder if they would be so eager if they knew the health disruptions of increased cervical and breast cancer rates. Who says there are increased rates of breast and cervical cancer? "They" do! Read the inserts.

> **Who says there are increased rates of breast and cervical cancer? "They" do! Read the inserts.**

In the past, we would share our message of health restoration each week, through a show I called "The Dr. Patrick Flynn Show." Viewers and patients sent us questions, so we could respond live and unscripted. It was a great outlet for many questions to be answered while getting the right information to people seeking answers. Here's a question I was asked, and then I will give you my response from one episode.

Hi Dr. Patrick, I am thirty-two years old. We have three children; my husband does not want anymore but I would not mind. He wants me on birth control. I started taking it and I don't feel good; I don't even feel like the same person! I've gained weight, I'm more emotional, but my husband said he will NOT use condoms. I've been following you for a long time and know it's not good for me and the more I research I do, I'm scared that I'm taking it. What research can I give him to convince him that I should not be on it? Also, he says it is fine because my OB said it was the best way to prevent another pregnancy.

First, we'll take this from the relationship side. Ladies, this is an interesting situation. Women will take care of their bodies. However, if their husband suggests for them to do something different, they will quickly do it. Typically, this is due to the deep need for connection and their desire to keep the peace in the relationship. You want research to convince him birth control is bad for you? Stop having sex with him. There's your research. Okay, that sounds aggressive, but hang in there with me. The research is everywhere. It's even on the package insert. His concern should be your health, not his convenience the few days a month you may be fertile. Unless he uses condoms, you aren't having sex. Ladies, understand, you have the control here.

> **Ladies, understand, you have the control here.**

I know I'll hear from Christian ladies out there, "But Doc, being a Christian woman, I just have to do what he wants and submit." Stop over-spiritualizing this situation. If he is putting you in an unhealthy place, you need to look at this more clearly. He may say he won't use condoms; the only option for him to be intimate with you is for you to put this unhealthy poison into your body. You need to rattle that boy's cage. You need to get a hold of him and tell him the man cave is closed. This isn't about submitting; this is about dysfunction and taking care of yourself. He needs to look at his relationship with his wife and not just his own needs. He may just want sex now, but he'll be getting a lot less of that if his wife gets sick with some of those known side effects. The dysfunction has to stop. This has to be about a healthy relationship and healthy bodies, together.

Often this isn't even a discussion. A man may have said he won't use condoms and she needs to take birth control. Because she desires that relationship, she caves. On the other hand, testosterone is a powerful motivator. If condoms are his only way to get to where he wants to go, he'll soon happily oblige. Ladies, trust me, you have more control over him than you think.

Here's another angle to this, many OB/GYNs may say this is the best thing for her to use to prevent pregnancy. It doesn't mean it's best for her body. Technically, there is an even better way to prevent pregnancy.

Abstinence. You'll have no kids if there is no sex. Frustrating? Sure, but you won't have to worry about pregnancy! It sounds silly and extreme, but honestly, the moment you tell him no, he'll go for a while without being intimate with you, but he'll quickly consider the use of condoms.

Looking at it from a health standpoint. Birth control is very detrimental to female health. It is an endocrine disrupter as defined by the EPA. It throws off the cycle and trust me, you'll end up with problems. Remember what medication does? It forces a response. Actually, medication by pharmacology definition is a non-lethal dose of a lethal substance.

Medication by pharmacology definition is a non-lethal dose of a lethal substance.

Many women don't feel like the same vibrant person she was before the birth control. Every time she looks at herself, she's probably bothered by the weight gain and her emotions are completely off. She's not going to be interested in sex. She's going to shut down because of all the changes going on in her body. Women, you are so self-conscious about your bodies. Most guys don't care about the subtle changes like weight gain in your body. But for you, this is huge and will disrupt your whole being, including your long-term health.

Keep your best interests at heart and say no to prescription birth control. If he becomes disrespectful and disruptive, my heart goes out to you for the kind of man you are dealing with. However, he doesn't control you, especially if it means causing you health problems.

I would hope that men would have their wives' best interest in mind, her health and physiology, her emotions, their relationship and even his own health. Because if they understood what birth control does, they wouldn't ask their ladies to put this into their bodies. Men, part of protecting her is protecting her health. If she thinks you'll stop loving her if she says no to endocrine-disrupting birth control, it's time for some serious reflection. Testosterone makes you a great protector—don't be afraid to use it.

Here's something few people realize about prescriptions, including birth control: that hormone shows up in your bodily fluids, not just your bloodstream. It is also in your saliva and your vaginal secretions. Ladies if you are on birth control, every time you kiss him or you have sex with him, he is exposed to the hormone. You are passing it to him. I have men come into the office and their estrogen and progesterone levels are way off. They ask me how it's possible. Is your wife on birth control? Well, then you're taking it too. When men realize this, and understand these synthetic hormones are also affecting his body and will create problems for him as well, they're quick to reconsider their stance on the matter!

What is one of the number one side effects of birth control? Cancer. Remember that insert of info from the pill packet? It lists all the disruptions it will cause in the woman's body, including

Ladies, if you are on birth control, every time you kiss him or have sex with him, he gets the hormone.

cancer. Sex with condoms becomes much less of a concern if and when a family is devastated by cancer.

Pills are not the only form of prescription birth control capable of causing such problems with hormones and health. IUDs and the patch are just as disruptive. You are not safe if you are using another endocrine disrupter form of birth control like the hormonal IUD, vaginal ring, implants, or the patch; all these things are destructive to hormones. Fortunately, there are non-hormonal options and more natural methods to prevent pregnancy. Timing a lady's cycle and either abstaining from intercourse or using condoms can be very effective. It does take more attention and is most effective when both partners are on board and attentive. Guys, here is yet another way you can help your lady and take some stress off her.

There are other natural methods to prevent pregnancy:

- Diaphragm
- Condoms
- Family planning

Not all women who are on birth control are taking it to prevent pregnancy. A study found 18% of women are taking the pill for non-contraceptive reasons. Many more relied on it for non-contraceptive purposes in addition to contraception. I wonder if the numbers would be the same if they all knew the consequences.

CHRISTY'S THOUGHTS

I was grateful when my mother told me that because of her own reproductive issues, she was not going to encourage us to get 'the pill' or any other drugs that doctors claimed would help. Even though my cystic acne was so bad, I got good at covering it up and many times avoided staying the night at friends' houses to avoid the embarrassment of them seeing me without it. Even though I got migraines in college, that was just the beginning of a seemingly downhill spiral of a hormone imbalance caused by stress that was slowly taking over my life. Even back then, I refused to believe that everything could be fixed with "the pill." Then came the cysts and the incredible pain -- and the only solution medical doctors had was drugs and surgery. I'm so thankful that I disagreed before I even knew better. Had I continued to go down the road they were recommending, I would not have had our four amazing girls!

Pharmaceutical companies are very good at marketing their products for a multitude of purposes, and birth control is no exception. They use what they know to address all kinds of concerns: acne, heavy periods, polycystic ovarian syndrome, endometriosis, migraines, and more. Each of those is regularly treated with a type of prescription birth control. You'll notice something interesting when you look at the inserts to see the potential negative effects. Some of them are the very ones they are treating you for.

You shouldn't have bad acne, horrible periods, or cysts and all that can come from disrupted hormones. If your hormones are out of proper ranges, it's not because you aren't taking a birth control pill. It's because there are other factors affecting your hormones and causing these symptoms. You can take all the medication you want to, but it doesn't fix the underlying

> **You can take all the medication you want, but it doesn't fix the underlying problems.**

problem. Thinking differently, getting your hormones tested and knowing how to best support your body to bring them back into proper ranges will help you see the clinical results you may have been hoping for from the prescription.

A study followed women in Denmark and other European countries and found those women using hormonal contraception had a significantly higher rate of developing depression. For young women, birth control pills are even gloomier. Those who were between the ages of fifteen and nineteen taking combination birth control pills were diagnosed with depression at a rate of 130%![1]
When we look at the risks and the impacts on hormonal balance, it's much bigger than just preventing pregnancy, or treating another condition. Prescription birth control is actually *causing* conditions we are working feverishly to stop! What's the easiest way to stop a condition though? Taking a different path—one that won't harm you to begin with.

1. Johansson, T., Larsen, S. Vinther, Bui, M., Ek, W.E., Karlsson, T, and Johansson, A. "Population-based Cohort Study of Oral Contraceptive Use and Risk of Depression." National Library of Medicine, June 12, 2023. https://www.ncbi.nlm.nih.gov/pmc/articles/PMC10294242/#ref31

CHAPTER 12

PUBERTY COMES TOO SOON.

Imagine a young girl visiting my office with her mom. Her feet swing underneath her chair as she reads a book, so the seven-year-old doesn't seem to hear us talking about precocious puberty—puberty at an early age. Her mom looks at me nervously as we sit in my office. Not only is this mom's niece experiencing this common, yet not normal phenomenon of breasts at age eight, but she hears other moms at the playground talking about it too. She's worried her daughter may be next. Someone told her it was because of the meat they ate; another person said it was because of the milk. The mom looks at me with a panicked look that I have seen time and time again from patients who have children, "Do I have to worry about my second grader and puberty? Isn't that something for middle school and high school? Is this normal?"

Having daughters, I get extremely serious about this. No, it's not normal, but we have been seeing the first signs of puberty happening at younger ages. I've seen this in as young as eight and nine-year-olds. Sometimes it's even kindergartners or younger. Who wants to teach their kindergartner about bras and how to tie their shoes at the same time? Not me. It already comes fast enough.

Over the past century, the age of first period has gone down worldwide from sixteen to under age thirteen.

If you go back in history, even fifty years ago, the average start of menstruation was between fifteen and sixteen years old. If you look at Biblical times, the Bible is such great documentation of history, most people were married and sometimes having kids right after menstruation began. Could you imagine if your daughter had her cycle at ten years old? Go back in history and with menstruation starting at fifteen, sixteen, or even seventeen, these

151

young women were almost adults already. What has changed to cause early development?

What used to happen in the late teens, and a signal it was time to be married, is now happening too soon. Who would be ready to marry off their eight-year-old? I want them to have more time for playgrounds, doll houses, and all the normal childhood experiences. Over the past century, the age of a first period has gone down worldwide from sixteen to under age thirteen. We are also seeing increased incidents of precocious puberty. This is when very young girls are experiencing puberty outside the normal window. What causes early puberty?

A common thought is that this is controlled by genetics; however, that's not the case. Our genome has not changed. The purpose of genetics is to keep your body normal, to support life. When you are born your genes make sure you develop to a healthy and normal state. If there is disruption during development, you can see some changes, but genes are not the determining factor here. Disruption to genes may be. What causes disruption to genetic expression? Stressors in the form of toxins, traumas, and thoughts.

What triggers puberty to begin? As we've learned, female cycles are more complicated than male cycles, puberty is no different. Do you know what else is complicated? Our modern environment. The only thing that causes a young girl to go from childhood to young womanhood is estrogens levels starting to rise. Estrogens can come from any number of places, including food and environment. If they are forced synthetically (prescriptions) or introduced to your body through other means, your genes and endocrine system will respond to that environment. Once you have induced puberty though, there is no going back.

What in our environment is leading to estrogens exposure to increase? We see the impacts of rising estrogens easily on young girls, but the same increased levels of estrogen are impacting us all. Making changes for our daughters is important, but we also want to make them for ourselves.

The meat and hormone issues are very well known and well documented—we'll look at that first.

They put the hormones into the cow to increase the growth rate and the mass of that animal. If you go back 200-300 years ago, the only people who ate muscle meat were the peasants, the slaves, and people of lower social statuses. Organ meats were the delicacy. The king wouldn't eat muscle meat. What changed? If you talk to a young person about organ meat, they freak out. Years ago, Grandma's house had liver paste. She happily served it, and we happily sat there eating heart, liver, kidney, and tongue.

The shift came when the farming industry recognized they couldn't increase production of organs at a high rate, but they could increase muscle meat. Now instead of grass feeding livestock, we're grain feeding them, which makes them grow bigger and faster. The food industry has come to value speed, convenience, and quantity. This is as a result of a number of influences, but the obvious result is a clear decline in quality. I get people who say, "Doc, healthy food is so expensive." Now that's opening the door to an entirely new conversation, but the question I usually ask then is: "Do you ever wonder why other food can be so cheap?" Most of it is something closer to a food-like product, not actual food.

The industry has focused on getting the animal to be larger, to weigh more so they can sell more as quickly as possible. This makes sense for them as a business—more product equals more sales! I understand! But the other side of the conversation is this: If you ingest the synthetic hormones added to foods, you're going to affect your hormones. So yes, meat could be one contributing factor, but it's not the only thing. Let's be clear, I am not saying to quit eating meat. I'm saying eat meat from a good source. Ask a local organic farmer what they feed their cows and buy half a cow. It's cheaper, healthier, and supports local industry!

There are many other triggers of precocious puberty. If there is an introduction of hormones, synthetic or natural, into any food source, it can induce early maturation and puberty. Xenoestrogens (chemicals that mimic the structure of estrogens) from all sources including pesticides, fertilizers, industrial chemicals, plastics (BPA and phthalates) can affect your body and hormone levels.

Do you know what the number one source for everyone—male, female, and child—to come in contact with hormones? It's not meat. The number one source of hormone introduction to the human body comes from city water.

Years ago, I went to see my sister in Spokane, Washington. We went to the gorgeous river. Right next to it was a water treatment facility. They're sucking the water and cleaning it out and pushing it back into the system. When we drove by, I pointed out to my sister that there's no filtration. Well, there's filtration, but here's what's happening. Water is treated for mineral content—anything that is naturally occurring in nature is treated and filtered in the plant. Things like sulfur and iron. If you've ever been somewhere with high sulfur in the water, you appreciate how great that filtration is! What's not filtered however, are chemicals.

When a woman who takes birth control pills pees, it goes into the water system and gets recycled back. Water treatment facilities don't have the type of filtration necessary to get prescription drugs back out of the system. With the increasing number of prescription drugs and synthetic hormones getting flushed into the system, this is a growing issue. At a municipal level, getting the filtration in place to address this is cost-prohibitive to say the least. However, you can easily add filtration to your home! The alternative, if you do not have proper water filtration in your home, you are exposed to everyone else's synthetic hormones in your showers, your cooking, and your drinking water.

Meat and water are two major contributors to early puberty. There are many other things considered endocrine disruptors that can also cause estrogens levels to rise. Many of them we come into contact with daily. The heavy metals in dental fillings, plastic water bottles and food storage, soft plastic toys and vinyl, metal cans for canned food, household cleaners and fragrances, flame retardants on children's pajamas, and other household products all contain endocrine disruptors that can affect reproductive hormones.

Here's an interesting one—one that seems indirect but isn't. You know what else can impact the onset of puberty? Whether your child plays outside or not. Children who are inside all the time playing video games or watching T.V. are more often less physically active. Physical activity is key to preventing obesity. According to the CDC, 22% of children ages 12-19 are obese.[1] This is important because estrogens are stored in fat. Studies have shown, girls who are obese will typically get their first period a year earlier than those who are not. Studies have shown obese boys will have a later start of puberty which could be because of greater estrogens levels.

Another reason to get your kids outside—they need vitamin D. Vitamin D is a vital hormone to keep the body functioning optimally. Studies have shown a link between vitamin D deficiency and early puberty. Girls closer to the equator will have a later start than those further away who don't see the sun as much. That's not good. One study showed girls who were vitamin D deficient were twice as likely to get their period early than those who had plenty of vitamin D.

> **Studies have shown a link between vitamin D deficiency and early puberty.**

1. Centers for Disease Control and Prevention. (2022, May 17). Childhood obesity facts. Centers for Disease Control and Prevention. https://www.cdc.gov/obesity/data/childhood.html#:~:text=For%20children%20and%20adolescents%20aged,to%2019%2Dyear%2Dolds.

CHRISTY'S THOUGHTS

We have a rule in our house we recently started. If anyone wants to watch TV, everybody has to do 10 pushups! It's just a fun way to get everyone active before enjoying some screen time. All the kids got into it. In fact, the younger girls are usually are the ones to get everyone together so they can watch something! Limiting the screen time is also important. Many people say they see positive behavior and attitude changes almost immediately. This is a way to get that extra movement in, even if you've already limited screen time. Building a healthy habit around a sedentary one is a good start. And it gets the whole family together!

During the summer, we want them outside as much as possible. From weeding or harvesting in the garden, to washing and preparing the produce, our girls are involved from seed to feed. We have so many life lesson discussions in our garden as we pull weeds (which can also be correlated to bad habits or thoughts!) and tending to plants so they can grow healthy!

Getting kids outside, moving, getting vitamin D, grounding -- all are so beneficial for their health in so many ways! It's easy, free, and builds such good life habits.

There are multiple things that can drive up estrogens levels. Remember, the body is like a Swiss watch. Like we have talked about, the only thing to cause the change from child to young womanhood are estrogens levels increasing. If they are forced artificially, your gene system will respond to the environment and bring on puberty. There is no reversing this effect.

So yes, we are looking at the issue of breasts developing much earlier in girls. There are a number of things we can do to address this. The mother at the beginning of the chapter was right. The meat source is possibly one of the causes due to the hormones that have been injected into that animal. This can be a simple change—meat without hormones is becoming more and more readily available as we learn the impact of those synthetics.

However, some of the other exposures to hormones through diet may need to be addressed. Does she need to worry because her niece is experiencing this and they are related? No, this is not a genetic issue. Your genes respond to help you to live the longest and healthiest life possible. You are not genetically programmed to suffer or to be sick.

It seems like a lot. There are a variety of triggers. We can't blame one thing or take a pill to get our desired outcome. But I'm excited to share this information with you because there are so many things you CAN do. There is a lot we can control if we take the time. We can clean it up—starting at home. Then in our communities—for our daughters, sons, and ourselves.

It's worth the time. Time is precious, especially when it's time to be a kid. As the father of four girls, I know it goes fast. They deserve this

> **You are not genetically programmed to suffer or be sick.**

time to swing their legs under their chair, laugh, and be carefree. They should not worry about our conversations about puberty. It all comes soon enough.

CHAPTER 13

THE "M" WORD.

Menopause is considered a bad word by many women. Most women cringe and fear the experience even before they enter this natural process. There aren't many women throwing parties for this transition in their life. But what if I told you women do not have to experience the difficult "symptoms" of menopause that you've likely heard about? First, let's understand what menopause is and what it isn't.

When you say the word menopause to a woman, do they think healthy, vital, and sexual right away? No. They think vaginal dryness, period problems, night sweats. That's not menopause. If you have any of these problems, I agree they're common, I want you to know that these symptoms are actually a sign you're hormones have been affected and are outside of optimal ranges. Menopause doesn't and shouldn't have to be that way.

Standard medical thinking and approach treats menopause like an unavoidable syndrome for women. The inevitable monster that is bound to rough you up any time after fifty years old. It's waiting for you, and it's just the way it is.

For a guy, we hit puberty, then we die.

It's exclusive to women, and very different from anything a man experiences. For a guy, we hit puberty and then we die. That's about it, if we keep ourselves healthy.

The largest medical establishment in the country is Mayo Clinic. Mayo had a definition for menopause on their website that illustrates why many women are likely confused and scared for this transition. Here's the Mayo Clinic definition:

Menopause is defined as occurring 12 months after your last menstrual period and marks the end of the menstrual cycles. Menopause can happen in your 40s or 50s with the average American woman beginning at age 51.

Ladies, if you go through menopause in your forties, that's alright, just get your hormone levels tested to be sure that is what is really happening. So far, we're doing great with this definition.

Menopause is a natural biological process. Although it also ends fertility, you can stay healthy, vital, and sexual. Some women feel relieved because they no longer worry about pregnancy.

They're correct. Everything Mayo Clinic said to that point is perfect. But there's a disconnect. If I were to walk up to a woman and tell her, "Menopause keeps you healthy, vital, and sexual," they'd look at me, laugh, and ask, "What planet are you from?"

Here's why. Mayo's next paragraph, after that perfect definition, is what women actually identify menopause with. Even so, the physical symptoms such as hot flashes, and emotional symptoms of menopause may disrupt your sleep, lower energy and for some women trigger anxiety and feelings of sadness and loss.

This is where the confusion comes in. How can you be healthy, vital, and sexual with that list of symptoms? This is where traditional medicine is limited in their perspective. Everything they've been taught—and therefore teach—is correct, but what they don't have is the thinking that would allow them to support hormone levels and prevent those symptoms. Menopause is a natural biological state and process, but it doesn't have to be miserable or medicated. Once, while I was teaching this subject to our audience, I noticed that Mayo updated their definition—sadly, they removed the part about staying healthy, vital, and sexual.

I had a sixty-four-year-old woman come in to see me. Her primary complaint was how she was suffering so badly from menopause symptoms. Guess what my first question was. Have you ever had your hormones tested? I wanted her to say it out loud, so she could hear it herself. You already know her answer. Nope. I tested her hormones, and they were devastatingly bad. We had discovered what was causing the fire and supported her hormones back to their proper levels and retested.

The next time I saw her our conversation went like this, "Doc, I'm doing so awesome, I feel amazing. I feel healthy, vital, and sexual!"

To which I replied, "Thank goodness I got rid of your menopause!"

She looked at me like I had grown a second head. I knew right away she had caught what I had said. I didn't get rid of her menopause! Menopause is a normal state of life if you live long enough. The only way for a woman to avoid it is to not reach that age in life.

It's so common for women to have a long list of symptoms they associate with menopause: irregular periods, hot flashes, vaginal dryness, night sweats, mood changes, weight gain, thinning hair, breast fullness, they believe those symptoms are menopause. This is not menopause; your hormone levels are off. Just because the symptoms are so common, women have accepted it as normal. Don't confuse common with normal. Is PMS normal? If it is, why is it called a "syndrome"?

When The Wellness Way doctors come along and talk about hormones and the basic biology of this transition, all of a sudden it makes sense for most women. It doesn't matter which Wellness Way clinic across the country you go to, or which doctor you see there, we all look at it from the same perspective. The body doesn't make mistakes. If women go through those symptoms, it's a signal their bodies are struggling as they are going through the change.

Our thinking is different, and our testing approach is different. We get a complete picture of what is going on and start to find out what is throwing those hormones off so that we can help women live in that healthy, vital, sexual state of menopause. Western medicine can address the symptoms with synthetic hormones. Yes, the

> **The first step is changing the way you think about menopause and the way you approach health care.**

synthetic hormone works to relieve the symptoms, but the side effect is often cancer. That's not a fair trade.

I'm sure some jaws will drop here, but I wish menopause for my wife. We have our four beautiful babies, and we've decided not to have anymore. I wish my wife could just go through menopause so she wouldn't have to deal with her cycle anymore. Does that sound like something any other man would wish for his wife if menopause were truly a horrible event? It is so much easier to keep a woman's hormones healthy and normal when she isn't cycling. A menopausal woman's hormone cycle isn't any different than a guy's really, it's just a flat line that's easy to keep right where it should be.

I had the blessing of helping my mom through this transition. Many people ask me what I did to help her. Well, first they ask me if I like taking care of my mom, especially through menopause. Yes! I want my mom to be healthy. I ran specific tests on her based on what I knew about her. There are multiple test options; blood, saliva, and urine. It depends on the woman and her situation. Each woman is unique and needs to be approached as such, not as a standard procedure. Based on her results there were many options to help her, and I can happily tell you her menopause experience was *normal*, not common.

The first step is changing the way you think about menopause and the way you approach your health care. If you took one of the test results I ran to a medical doctor, he'd look at the test from the perspective of which prescription for medication he could write for you. I appreciate that – he's trying to save you from the discomfort! What different thinking allows you to do, however, is rebuild your house, so you aren't dependent on a synthetic hormone or worse yet, a psychiatric drug for the rest of your life. You can not only survive menopause but thrive and live a life that is healthy, vital, and sexual. Your body was created to go through menopause as a healthy stage of life.

PART 3

HOPE RESTORED.

CHAPTER 14

MAKE IMMUNE SYSTEMS STRONG AGAIN.

It's so good, I'll say it again. Make Immune Systems Strong Again! It was a campaign we ran at The Wellness Way clinics during the COVID years. It blew everyone away, so many people felt empowered with this message and took back control of their health, even talk to doctors and family members when they dared to disagree. Why did this message resonate with so many people? Because we've done so much to affect their immune responses and have contributed to more and more health concerns! How?

Think back to when you were a child, and you might feel under the weather, a little tickle in your throat, a runny nose, a bit icky. What was your parents' first reaction? I'm going to guess they ran you to the doctor, filled prescriptions, and had bottles of acetaminophen and decongestant near your bedside. If you are a bit older or you had the privilege of being raised around grandparents, what would they have done? Tell you to stay in bed, drink fluids, make chicken soup, and support your body to ride it out. Today, the general population is so scared of a cold or simple childhood illness that the body is designed to fight that it is assumed we couldn't possibly fight it without pharmaceutical intervention. Let me say this, there is no condition due to a lack of pharmaceuticals. We aren't prescription deficient!

> **Let me say this, there is no condition due to lack of pharmaceuticals. We aren't prescription deficient.**

Think about this, how many antibacterial products are on the market today? Everything is antibacterial! But did you know that you need the helpful bacteria that is supposed to live on your skin? Guess which bacteria these products kill? All of them! Antibacterial soap isn't intelligent. It doesn't know which bacteria to kill and which to allow to thrive. Your immune response is dependent on that first line of defense. If you wipe that out, you should be worried about every bacterium you come in contact with!

Think about how kids were once encouraged to get outside and get dirty. Today we are so focused on daily baths, constant handwashing, making sure there is hand sanitizer at every turn, and sterilizing everything. Immune responses don't stand a chance of actually being developed and strengthened. They are born at one level and then beaten down from the beginning!

Consider this, when a baby is born in a hospital, within hours, on day one of a child's life, it is common to flood their little bodies with medications from vaccines for illnesses to vitamin K in the name of helping them to be healthy. Do you know what they don't do before they do that to each infant? Test their immune response to see if this is even beneficial to them. Their immune responses, liver, and detox pathways, nothing is prepared for the whole bunch of things we inject into them. I have to wonder; what kind of nursery is that hospital running if the Hepatitis B vaccine is given on day one? That is a condition that most commonly affects IV drug users and prostitutes. I'm thinking we should be asking bigger questions if that is one thing we do across the board at every hospital across the U.S. for every baby. Oh wait. That's all been documented, too. You'll have to dig deeper than the pretty pastel sheet the nurse handed you as they injected your baby.

I disagree that all vaccines are safe and effective, that they offer maximum benefits to the immune response, and that they are the best approach to many illnesses. Clearly, I disagree with the CDC's childhood vaccine schedule. You know what else I disagree with? How we've conditioned people to believe they can't possibly support their innate immune response. What is the innate immune response? Let me share some insights to not only explain that but also why making immune systems strong again is a different perspective.

CHRISTY'S THOUGHTS

I discovered that many of my health issues stemmed from immune issues. The hormonal issues were secondary and downstream from these challenges that started as immune concerns. In fact, I knew I had vaccine injuries; I had connected the dots. As a result, I had decided in college that I wouldn't be vaccinating my children. I had met children who weren't vaccinated and was able to see an amazing difference between them and other vaccinated children. I knew what I wanted for my children. It wasn't until I met Patrick, and he started explaining why I was seeing the difference, and how the vaccines affected the body that I truly understood. I was so excited to have someone to raise children with who agreed with me on this! I continued to learn from other vocal doctors and pioneers on this very controversial topic. Today, we have 4 very healthy, unvaccinated daughters. And I don't regret a minute of that decision!

The steps I took to take care of my immune response between and during each pregnancy led to healthy babies, to the point where our youngest gets through everything so quickly! Mommas, take care of your immune response, and build your baby's! By sharing our story and other people's stories, we can help them have different outcomes and set their families up for health success. Building the support system The Wellness Way provides allows others to make those bold decisions confidently.

THE INNATE AND THE ADAPTIVE — A DYNAMIC DUO!

Let's start with something that I know is going to blow your mind. Ready? Most everything we know about the immune system changes every year as we discover and uncover more about it. From textbooks used in medical schools to scientific research, most of it changes. Why? There are so many organs and cells that make up this intricate response that it's almost unfair to call it a system. That is why I prefer to call it the immune response. Each person's personal history, genetic information, and exposure to the environment will impact how they react. It is hard to predict how one person's immune response is going to react compared to another. There will be similarities, but some people react very differently. Most all books, research, and papers are observations. And to think, this is what governed how our families saw each other for holidays during COVID. Well, not my family, but many others.

You know how I like to help boil down complicated concepts and make them easy to understand? I think when that is the situation, you can make better decisions and not live in fear. Let's take a look at the immune response from a different perspective.

Imagine that there is a constant battle going on inside and outside of your body. You are constantly facing toxins and biotoxins (ones made from living things). But don't fear! The good news is that your body was designed to handle those potentially harmful things!

Let's consider some immune responses and what your body is doing. Just remember, the body is always trying to adapt to internal and external factors. The first step of your immune response is your barrier. What is your biggest barrier? Your skin! Your skin produces enzymes to protect you from bacteria and viruses. The skin in your nose, mouth, and ears also helps produce these protective enzymes so that those proteins are taken care of quickly. This is why when you come in contact with something, your nose or throat may burn, it's doing its job and defending against the invading proteins. Your body knows how to respond! Remember that anti-bacterial soap and hand sanitizer we talked about earlier? It's destroying those enzymes!

When you were born, you were created with an innate immune response to keep you alive. Your mom's immune response is handed down to you at birth. White blood cells and interferons are protective immune cells you are born with so that you can get a healthy start in life. These little macrophages, little dendritic cells, will actually eat up those bacteria and virus proteins and spit them back out.

What happens every September? Your child goes to school and, after a few days or weeks, comes home with the sniffles. Why? Schools are like huge Petri dishes! Each one of those kids is bringing in new viruses and bacteria to be spread around. Those mucous membranes go to work to encapsulate those foreign proteins, and boogery noses and sore throats circulate through that classroom. Why? Each of those little innate immune responses is protecting and adapting. Adapting to what? The environment and the "bugs" they are being exposed to. Does that make sense? When your child has a runny nose or a sore throat, they aren't sick. That is a very healthy immune response taking care of business!

Do they feel a bit crummy? Sure! Do they need decongestants and fever suppressors? No! If you give it to them, you are interfering in the way of that immune response and the healthy adaptation to new, foreign proteins! Those symptoms we see, from runny noses to coughs are designed to push the virus out. The fever is the body waging war and fighting off the virus that can't survive the increase in temperature. Do we, as parents, feel bad for them? Sure, because they feel crummy. But if you look at it from a different perspective, you can be excited that their body is adapting and doing exactly what it is designed to do!

If you allow kids to go through those immune building responses, you set them up for a better response later in life.

If you allow kids to go through those immune building responses, you set them up for a better response later in life. To be honest, I feel bad for kids who are totally sheltered from everything and not allowed to build that response. They are the ones whose bodies may not be prepared later in life for some of the more serious conditions they may face.

I know what you might be thinking. There are parents who are so excited to get their kids exposed to everything. They hear of chickenpox and are ready to share spoons and bathtubs so that their kids are exposed. They think then they'll have immunity and be set for life. Actually, only if those memory cells (adaptive immune system) are prepared to handle it and the response is prepared...but here's something to think about. From chickenpox to COVID, that response is so unique to the person. I agree, if kids can go through an infection naturally and handle it, they are better set up for the future. But what if their bodies aren't prepared for that battle? That's a bad day!

There's another myth we need to bust. This whole notion of "boosting" immune systems.

There's another myth we need to bust. This whole notion of "boosting" immune systems. First of all, you've heard my take on immune systems. Second, boosting is quite a weird narrative to me. Let me explain. The only way I can see "boosting" is giving it extra, making it work harder. Isn't that like an autoimmune condition or infection where the immune response is heightened and constantly triggering? In reality, what we can do is support the immune response. Support the organs, the bone marrow which produces some of the immune cells, take the extra stress off the body, feed and nourish it with what it needs to produce a good, healthy response when the time is right.

Here is one of the best ways to think about supporting your immune response. What if you could set your body up for the best success, the best clinical results, even for things like seasonal allergies and a common cold? The innate immune response can be absolutely messed up by deficiencies and toxicities. Nutritional deficiencies mean the body doesn't have the fuel to run the engine of your immune response. You wouldn't expect your car to move without the proper fuel. Why are you expecting it from something much more intricate like your body?

Remember back toward the beginning when we talked about the 3Ts – traumas, toxins, and thoughts? Each of those has a dramatic effect on the immune response. One area we find that helps people have the best results nearly immediately is one very specific and emotional one. Food allergies. Food allergies can cause a toxic situation in the body. Remember my story early on in the book? Eggs were (and still are) my kryptonite! Once I was aware of how stimulated they caused my immune response to be, I was able to take back control of my health and even my mindset.

If you are constantly eating something your body has to wage war on, you are triggering IgG, IgA and IgE antibodies. We're all familiar with IgE, think "emergency" like anaphylaxis, swelling, or even death. Those IgGs can be less obvious. Either way an immune response is happening. How can we tell? Run a panel to see if you are responding. Is it possible? Yes. We do it every day, hundreds of times a day, across the U.S. and around the world and help people find those answers. But that's not the only testing tool we have in our toolbox. Keep reading.

CHARLIE'S STORY

When I was about 27 years old and maybe two years into practice, I met a guy who would change my practice forever. Let's call this guy Charlie.

Let me tell you the story. It's an emotional story. It's actually sometimes very difficult to tell because, unlike many of my stories, this one didn't have a happy ending. But the unhappy ending led to the transformation of hundreds of thousands of lives.

I was taking care of this wonderful woman that came in for hormone issues, and she was getting great clinical results. One day when she came in, she said, "Doc, I'd really like you meet my brother." I said, "Sure, cool." Most doctors early on know that their patient base comes from referrals, so I always appreciate it when patients refer friends and family. She told me he was in from California and would like to see me. I was thinking that he was going to come to see me because he had testosterone problems or some healthcare problems, so I asked her what was going on with him.

I remember it like it was yesterday. She said, "He has AIDS." I worked hard to keep my face stone straight. But in my head, I was like, *holy man!* I learned about HIV and AIDS in school, not to the extent of what to do with it or anything like that because that's a whole other topic. I'm going to be very upfront and honest with you I was a bit thrown and wondering things like, *Can I hug him? Can I shake his hand? What if he sneezes on me? Am I going to get AIDS? I'm not joking.* I was just 27 years old, naive as hell, and worried about getting AIDS myself. So, I had to ask myself, *What do I do now?* I was sort of nervous about meeting him, kind of like many people were during the COVID days, scared to come in contact.

I just looked at her and told her I'd be excited to see him. But inside, I was trembling and wondering what the heck I was going to do. Then I slowed down for a minute and worked through it. All right, HIV, there's a change in the immune response that is causing a problem. Now, I wasn't there to deal with his condition, I was thinking I would like to see his immune labs and see what I can do to support his body.

I love the immune response and I continue to take post-graduate classes to this day. The first thing I did was ask if he had any labs. Of course, they figured he'd had so many tests run they had plenty to share. It's kind of similar to Christy's story, where they thought they had all the proper testing done, but it was so incomplete.

> **They *thought* they had all the proper testing done, but it was so incomplete.**

I started thinking critically and asked myself, How do I actually even test an HIV or AIDS patient? I got his labs that he'd had run before he came to see me. There were very specific things they were looking at, but the markers they were looking at covered such a minimal part of his immune response. He had tests every two weeks for his white blood cell count. Looking at the numbers, I could tell things were going downhill. I knew there had to be more than that. I knew there were more immune cells than that that had to be checked. And, no joke, I was trying to come up with a way, with some markers we could use to actually get a good, comprehensive test on him. All the research I was finding was talking about CD4 cells and CD8 cells.

So I started to research a little bit more about it. Lymphocytes are a type of white blood cell in your immune response. This test I was studying looks at two of them. The CD4 and CD8. CD4 cells lead the fight against infections. CD8 cells can kill cancer cells and other invaders. If you know anything about HIV, the HIV virus will actually attach to CD4 cells and destroy them. If you ever notice, people usually don't die from a virus. They usually die from a secondary infection. It's why they give antibiotics to people who have a virus. It doesn't affect the virus. They use it because the majority of people actually die from bacteria. That's what the antibiotic was for. Now that you know a bit more, what if we supported the body to actually fight the virus? Would we have to worry about a secondary infection so much? The virus actually just weakens sick people to the point that the bacterium can kill pretty quickly.

I was thumbing through his stuff, and realized he hadn't had CD4 cells tested in a long time. He just had markers for general white blood cell count but no specifics, which in this case and many others, makes a big difference! It reminded me of when I had first seen Christy's tests for her estrogens. Where's all the rest of them? Their testing for the immune response was incomplete. For an immune response condition.

Remember how I said above that HIV affects the CD4 cells? Viruses need you. Let me say that again. Any virus on this planet, from influenza to Corona, to SARS, to HIV, needs you. They need your DNA, they need your RNA, they need your cells. They cannot replicate by themselves. That's why they're, by nature, parasitic. So, with HIV, your number of CD4 cells will drop, and the lack of CD8s leads to more frequent infections. In that case, people can get a secondary infection, and that's what most die from. Does it make better sense now?

If you look at cancer, heart disease, and all major diseases, do you understand that many people actually die from infection in the hospital? But it's listed as heart disease. It's listed as cancer. People often say, "They got pneumonia and died." Well, there's pneumonia and viruses everywhere. Do you understand? No joke. Viruses are by far the most abundant thing on the planet. Do you know if you take roughly one liter to a gallon of ocean water, there's like a billion viruses in that one sample? Do you understand you can't get away from them? There are viruses all around us that we don't even know exist yet. Yet we walk around in fear of one specific one or another. I'd walk around in fear if my CD4 and CD8 cells were low! But I don't, and I'll tell you why in a bit.

I put together a test for Charlie. The test looked at the ratio of CD4 and CD8 cells and more. Listen closely, this right here can change the direction of your life. The ratio tells your healthcare provider how strong your immune response is. Let me say that again. The ratio tells your healthcare provider how well your body is functioning to protect itself, this can affect how you respond to a virus. If you had that knowledge, would you be afraid of every virus that goes around? Would you be better equipped to take care of your more fragile family members?

So, I told Charlie I'd like to get some blood work done and we got the labs set. You could tell he was not doing well. He was pale, coughing a lot, and physically weak, but was also looking for any kind of help. After our appointment, he went and visited family in town for a little bit. Several days after that, he went back home to California, and died shortly after.

So, I sat there. Upset. Frustrated. Sad for the family. I sat there and thought, *What if I could have got this information to him a year ago?* Could I guarantee that I would be telling a different story, that he would have lived? No, I can't.

But what if we could have got information and stuff to him before? And that's when I had my lightbulb moment. Because I got his labs back.

After looking at all the labs, looking at all the testing, looking at all the immune response, guess what. Specific immune markers were really low. There is research to show that you can support the body during these deficient states to help it come back to a more normal state.

While I couldn't get answers in time to help Charlie, what I learned from meeting him and digging deeper, trying to help him, has led to a test that has helped so many people take a look at their immune response so that they could make better decisions regarding their health and healthcare options. I don't live in fear. I know how strong my immune response and each of my family members is.

There is someone whose story I'd like you to hear. She is like a little sister to me, and one of medical providers whom I trust from that world. Nicole works at our Green Bay location. Her story follows here, and she is the guest author for our next chapter. Wait till you hear this! I'm sure you'll get so much hope just hearing from her.

NICOLE'S STORY

So many things are clearer with hindsight. If you asked my younger version if I'd ever thought I'd be here, I'd probably have laughed you out of the room. In fact, when I first came to The Wellness Way, my friends and family did laugh at me, never believing I'd be the "healthy/crunchy one". And yet, there is nowhere else I could be to carry out what I believe is my God-given mission. It just took an interesting path to get here. At specific times in my story, nothing made sense. Looking back, today, it all makes sense.

Since puberty at age 11, I have struggled with my periods. They were regular in terms of time, but they were also painful, leading to missed school. My periods were so heavy it led to severe anemia…I'll never forget passing out while standing on the choir risers because I literally couldn't see straight as my brain was starving of oxygen. Clearly, this wasn't normal, so my mom took me to many specialists, where I earned my first colonoscopy at just twelve years old to find the source of low iron levels. These specialists never found the cause of the anemia and why I would frequently pass out…it seemed impossible that it could be simply just from terrible, awful, heavy periods. Looking back, it looks so obvious, yet never seemed to be part of the hypotheses they'd throw at me.

My mom, being the good mother she was, just desperately trying to help her girl, approved the use of birth control to help steady my period. I did find some relief for the seven years that I was on it. When I left for college and started planning a wedding, I knew that my periods were inconsistent. I wanted to have a more regular life and let my body adjust and find a normal rhythm. I knew this would take some time so 6 months before my husband and I got married, I went off birth control to help my body find it's natural way before we would decide to start a family. Deep down, I think that I just was afraid, that perhaps I was broken, and didn't want to prevent a pregnancy, if God decided to bless me with a child.

My biggest fear was that I wouldn't be able to have kids.

I remember distinctly going on a mission trip in high school, and during a team-building exercise we went around the circle and shared our biggest fears. Many of the kids mentioned normal things like heights, spiders, snakes, the dark. My biggest fear was that I wouldn't be able to have kids. I was so certain that I was broken and that this wouldn't be in the cards for me, that when we were going through pre-marital counseling, I had convinced myself I didn't want kids. I think it was a defense mechanism. I convinced myself that if I didn't want children, it would soften the blow when a doctor might one day tell me that

I couldn't. Through that pre-marital counseling, I realized that I really did want kids, I was just too afraid to admit it. It was a goal I didn't want to fail at. As someone who is an "achiever" at heart, and very goal-driven, it scared me that this may be something about myself that I wasn't truly in control of. I didn't want to "fail" at the whole "being a woman" thing.

After stopping the birth control, I went months without getting a period. I was a virgin at the time, but I was convinced I had somehow gotten pregnant. I had all those stupid thoughts that you've heard about. The ones virgins have about perhaps getting pregnant from a hot tub or public toilet…because it didn't make sense that I would go so long without one! Finally, it did make it's ugly appearance and it was incredibly painful and it would then be months before having another one.

I finally went to see a Nurse Practitioner about the issues. She did some further testing, and I was diagnosed with Polycystic Ovary Syndrome (PCOS). Because I had such irregular periods, they told me it would likely be very difficult for me to conceive. This news was devastating. My worst nightmare had come true. A challenge that intuitively, I guess I always knew would be something I'd face. I found out a few months before I was supposed to get married, and I was terrified to tell my fiancé that perhaps I couldn't be a mother and provide the family he desperately wanted.

"I don't know if I'm going to be able to have kids. Are you sure you still want to marry me even if this is something I can't give you?" I asked him. He was surprised but assured me that whatever it takes, we'd figure this out together. The reality that I might be unable to have children, that we may struggle to have a family, felt like a nightmare.

We started our marriage in this stage of not knowing what our future family would look like. During that first year of marriage while dealing with the diagnosis of PCOS, I gained 70 pounds. When we had been married two years, I was still in college, so we weren't actively trying to have a baby. Because I knew that the possibility existed that it would be difficult for

me to conceive, we decided we weren't going to prevent any
pregnancy with birth control. We decided that if it happens,
it happens. A baby would be God's gift to us. Reality was, all
these people around me were getting pregnant that didn't want
to be, and my heart grew jealous and bitter. I was having a
hard time processing our situation. We were married. We had a
good home for welcoming babies. Why wasn't this happening
for us? I went into a depression thinking parenthood was not a
part of our story.

One night I was just lying in bed and I started praying.
*"God, I do feel like I'm going to have a baby someday, but could you
give me a dream or a sign or something to help me get in the right
mindset if adoption is my future? Please, bring me some sort of
clarity. I'm afraid of the unknown."* That night I dreamed I was in
a dark room with my eyes closed, rubbing my belly and feeling
that distinct kick of a baby growing in the womb. I felt in my
dream that someone had said, "His name is Simon." I woke up
wondering what it meant. Simon is very specific and a name
I wouldn't normally have picked for a baby. However, God
has named a lot of people throughout history. I looked up the
meaning of the name Simon; He has heard. I was stunned. The
next month I found out I was pregnant with my son. Of course,
we named him Simon!

After Simon was born, I was still very overweight.
My doctor prescribed Metformin, a prescription often given to
people who have PCOS. It helps insulin resistance, a common
concern with PCOS. It gave me digestive upset. I never knew
when I would have random, urgent, uncontrollable diarrhea,
and it was awful. After a month, I stopped taking Metformin
and decided I was going to have to live with the situation and
deal with it. I felt like, at this time, God was whispering to me,
"get your body back to healthy, and the second one will come." I
tried everything. Exercising. Drinking meal replacement shakes.
Eating healthy. I was doing all I knew to do. You know the
standard to get your body healthy—diet and exercise. I lost 20
pounds on my own, but it was difficult.

While all of this was happening, I was struggling with an autoimmune condition that no one could identify. I had eczema all over my body. After I had Simon, the eczema got worse. One night, I cried myself to sleep. My body was on fire. My husband was draping wet towels all over me. It was the only thing that offered even a bit of soothing relief. I was a labor and delivery nurse at the time and had to sanitize my hands every time I walked in and out of a patient room. The sanitizer would burn my hands and rub them raw. I remember asking my rheumatologist if there was anything I could do besides steroids to address all of the eczema, and that it hurt my hands so much working as a nurse. His response was either I had to quit my job or move to Florida where I could have more access to available sunlight. Those were the options he gave me. So we started considering moving to Florida because tanning did seemed to help because of the Vitamin D benefits. I had all these things I was trying to piece together, and I just couldn't. When I was 23, I was diagnosed with Rheumatoid Arthritis. I was in my junior year of nursing school, and I could not write notes because it hurt my joints so badly. I got myself an iPad and laptop to do everything I could digitally. Holding a pencil and taking copious notes was way too much pain.

I was overweight. I had this terrible bleeding eczema all over my body. I couldn't hold a pen. I had tried everything. I had used steroids. I tried Chinese medicine. I tried silver. I tried every cream, essential oil, and potion I could find. If I thought it would help eczema, I bought it. I spent thousands of dollars. Some remedies might help for a short time, but if I ever went a day without it, the symptoms would creep right back. I was exercising and eating healthy, but not losing weight. I found a detox program online. I checked it out, since I'd heard a lot of people lose a lot of weight on detox, I bought it.

The program was a 21-day detox, where you take some supplements, and they tell you what to eat every single day. At the end of the detox, the end of the 3 weeks, I was finally seeing some relief for the first time in my life from the eczema. It was almost gone. It was interesting because I wasn't doing anything topically. I didn't realize it, I was just working on my gut and my insides. Two weeks later, I had a period for the first time in months. Two weeks after that, I conceived my daughter.

During pregnancy your immune system changes so things tend to go better for those with autoimmune challenges. If you have an autoimmune disease and fall pregnant, women feel AMAZING! After I had my daughter, I was thinking Okay, there is something to this detox thing.

As a nurse working in labor and delivery, I was used to the medical mindset and pharmacology practices. I was stuck with the mindset of taking a drug for a condition. I didn't like the drugs they gave me; often they made me feel worse, but I couldn't find anything else that would work. I thought I was stuck.

I remembered the eczema had gone away with the detox. I was starting to connect the dots. However, I felt like I couldn't be living in a state of detox all the time, that didn't seem right. I had questions, and was eager to learn more, so I went to a conference. The man who had created the program I had used was there. I asked him about the idea of living in a constant state of detox. He told me it was possible. There are ways to support your body through supplementation to keep the inflammation at bay. Inflammation. There was another dot. I did another detox and felt fantastic. This was the only time I'd lose weight quickly and the eczema would go away. I was doing research and found there was a connection between eczema and gut health. There's something to this gut health thing! I was determined to get healthy, and the pieces were coming together!

I've always been transparent about my journey on Facebook. One day, someone reached out to me and told me

I was doing research and found there was a connection between eczema and gut health.

about this gut protocol and invited me to do it with them. It was a five thousand-dollar program plus the supplements. I was desperate. While I was doing this gut healing program, someone else reached out to me and asked if I'd ever heard of Dr. Patrick and The Wellness Way. I was in the middle of the program. I had spent several thousand dollars on this gut thing; I was going to stick with it. They were relentless "he really makes the connections when he talks about your gut health, he talks about how it affects your hormones, inflammation, everything." All I could think was it's all connected! It's not just gut = eczema, it's gut = hormones and eczema and I have all these things going on. Maybe it all originates in my gut!

I was seeing some results from the gut protocol, but not like I wanted for how much I had paid. I called to set up an appointment with Dr. Patrick. I've never shared this publicly, but I was so miserable in my own body, I really sank into a deep depression, and even had some suicidal thoughts. I didn't want to live like this anymore, and I was desperate for answers as soon as humanly possible. I remember sitting in the waiting room thinking, Either these people are going to be a bunch of weirdos (and truly if steroids can't help me, surely lavender won't) and totally out there or there's going to be something to this. I'm about to find out. They

Either these people are a bunch of weirdos (and truly if steroids can't help me, surely lavendar won't), or there's going to be something to this. I'm about to find out.

took my x-rays and showed me the inflammation in my gut. Let me repeat that, they showed me the inflammation in my gut! Dots connected.

I talked with Dr. Patrick and told him my story. I had brought in my giant tub of supplements that I was taking. His response, "there's nothing wrong with these supplements but

181

how do you know they are the ones you need?" All I could say was, "I don't know, it's just part of the protocol." He showed me the problem with the protocol. It wasn't individualized to each person. That's why I wasn't getting the results I was looking for. He started to help me shift my mind and think differently.

There's nothing wrong with these supplements but how do you know they are the ones you need?

I went to the Inflammation Talk the next day. Finally, it clicked. The Wellness Way clinics offer Inflammation Talks every couple of weeks for new patients. This talk is the foundation and introduces new patients to their approach. Inflammation is the key to all sources of disease and dysfunction within the body. This is what I had been looking for. I had been researching for years trying to find answers and connect the dots between my gut, eczema, autoimmune, conditions and PCOS. I finally found someone who could put those connections together!

After the Inflammation Talk, I boldly approached Dr. Patrick. The only thing I could think was, if there's anything I am going to do, I have to work for this guy. I have to learn everything he knows. I said, "I don't know if you remember me. I was in as a new patient yesterday. I had mentioned that I am a nurse. Your Inflammation Talk opened my eyes. I finally get it. Women's hormones and autoimmune conditions are my passion; it's something I have struggled with. I really think this approach could apply to infertility for women across the country and I want to be the one they come to. Would you consider bringing me on board?" His response was quick, "Yes, come in for an interview." I was totally blown away. "REALLY?" I'm not typically that bold, but there was something inside me. I knew I couldn't leave without addressing it.

I went in for the interview. The timing was perfect. The clinic in Green Bay, Wisconsin, was looking for a nurse to help with the IV center. It was a great way to get trained and see what happens at The Wellness Way. My wellness journey began. I recognized the difference between The Wellness Way Approach and the medical model I had been trained in. The allopathic medical model sees a list of symptoms and comes up with a diagnosis to treat. They don't look at the whole picture. It didn't resonate with me that I'd have to live a life constantly relying on medication or supplements like others suggested. I felt like I should be able to fix it. Medication or supplements should be part-time. The Wellness Way looks at things differently and looks at people as individuals.

> **I recognized the difference between The Wellness Way Approach and the medical model I had been trained in.**

First, I properly tested my thyroid, hormone, and food allergies. My food allergy test was eye-opening. I discovered I had 42 food allergies. To this day, I have not had anyone come into the Green Bay clinic with more than me. I started eliminating those immediately. It was very difficult, but necessary. I started taking a few supplements to help with my gut, my iron deficiency, and to balance my hormones. Unlike a traditional PCOS patient, I had very low testosterone. A lot of the protocol used in the medical world wouldn't have worked for me; I wouldn't have known why if I hadn't gotten my hormones tested so thoroughly. Within a month of following this new approach, I got my period for the first time in months. It was the first normal period in my life. From then on, I would get it every single month. The first week I lost 10 pounds. I was 80 pounds overweight at that time. Within my first two months, I lost over 25 pounds and 60 pounds within the first 6 months. I was feeling like myself again. I had more vitality and energy. Within two months, my eczema was completely gone. I was a walking testimony to The Wellness Way Approach!

Everyone had told me I would have autoimmune conditions and take steroids for the rest of my life. Rheumatoid arthritis, eczema, weight, and PCOS were four different systems that were all broken. When I came to The Wellness Way, I realized they were connected; they weren't isolated instances. I started sharing my Wellness Way testimony with my friends and have become a great referral source. I soaked up everything I could about hormones and how to balance the body. When my husband and I decided we were ready, we conceived baby #3 the first time we tried. I believe this lifestyle is for everyone. But it takes perseverance, dedication, and discipline. You shouldn't have to take supplements or medication for the rest of your life. Your body can be whole, well, and free of conditions as long as you know and avoid your triggers.

My dreams and desires to reach as many people as I can are becoming reality. At The Wellness Way, we don't have specialties; everything within the body is connected. However, I have been able to build a practice around this very special focus. It is so much fun to help women find the contributing factors of their issues, and then address them and watch them feel so much better like I did. We've had people reach out from all over the world through the power of social media. Women from Switzerland, Argentina, Bhutan, Asia, England, and countless others have found answers.

Every time I share The Wellness Way message, I tell my patients, "You are not broken." A lot of times, when women are not able to conceive, it devastates them. It's part of their womanhood; they feel like they are broken. The reality is, your body is responding to your environment, we just have to figure out why and fix it. You were created to have babies if that is what you want! And NO woman is the exception to that rule.

CHAPTER 15

I DISAGREE THAT CANCER IS A LIFE SENTENCE.

With contributing author Nicole Saleske FNP-BC, APNP

Okay, so you've read my personal story and how I came to The Wellness Way. Several years have passed since I told that story for the original I Disagree book. Since that time, I went on to become an Advanced Practice Family Nurse Practitioner. One of the hardest things about nurse practitioner school was that I had to constantly take off my Wellness Way hat to think allopathically…a mindset I worked so hard to deprogram from my mind. I remember sometimes answering questions in exams knowing what answer they wanted me to say, when in reality I didn't even agree with any of the answers given to me on the multiple choice. But in the end, that helped me see everything from two totally different perspectives with the ability to coach my patients as to what they would hear from their medical, allopathic doctors, and why that methodology likely wouldn't lead to the discovery of the "why" behind their diagnosis, ever. You see, in school we aren't trained to ask for the "why." In NP school there are the "pillars" of our education: Human Assessment, Pathophysiology (how disease affects the body, not even 'physiology' how the body works), and Pharmacology. So basically, assess your patient, give their issue a name, and treat it with a drug. Beyond that, I wasn't trained in anything else on how to actually heal the body. (And news flash: you can't heal the body if you don't actually change what made it sick in the first place…you can only cover up symptoms – which isn't true healing…I digress).

In my spare time (just kidding, there wasn't any), I built a practice known for helping women and couples on their fertility journey. Of course, if you've come this far in the book, you know that it was simply taking a look at many factors and systems in the body to discover what was causing their bodies to adapt in what presented as infertility. In reality, we awakened the body's ability to do what it was designed to do – to procreate, by eliminating the triggers that were preventing it from doing so. I loved what I did in helping to bring forth life, that wouldn't be here otherwise, and help couples to meet their dream child. In 2020, when COVID hit the scene, I knew that I was prepared to take on even bigger challenges… I had another stirring in my heart that caused me to look at what The Wellness Way does and what I could offer to people.

I'll never forget, I was sitting in one of our conference rooms one Saturday with Dr. Patrick and a Wellness Way friend who happens to be a pharmacist, as we were preparing for our weekend show. I'm not the only one from the allopathic world The Wellness Way has inspired! We were discussing the new mRNA vaccines for COVID and were dissecting the science behind it and predicting what may be on the horizon as the next health crisis wave and future challenges. It was crystal clear, like writing on the wall. It became glaringly obvious that soon we would witness an incredible wave of autoimmune conditions and cancer. I knew it in my heart, and I felt a calling on my soul. I felt like God had told me in that moment, cancer is coming, be prepared. This was the new direction for my practice. I told Dr. Patrick this and laid out a plan. It would require some additional education and certifications, that would be an investment. He knew instantly that I was on to something big, then tossed me his credit card and told me to get out of there and get to work. Now, in true Wellness Way fashion, we took the teachings from what I learned about the Metabolic Approach to Cancer from Dr. Nasha Winters and crafted a program that people from all over the U.S. are reaching out to and seeking solutions and guidance for their cancer journey.

WAIT, WHY CANCER?

Let me add a bit to the story you just read. I think it will fill in a few blanks. Picture it, an enthusiastic nursing student waiting tables at Buffalo Wild Wings. Every year I would raise money for St. Jude's Children's Hospital in Memphis as part of our fundraising efforts in September. They would hold contests to see which servers could get the most donations. Being competitive in nature, I wouldn't just rise to the occasion to raise money…I blew everyone else out of the water! I was enthralled by the vision of their founder, Danny Thomas. Together, we (donators, families, researchers, and medical staff) would eradicate childhood cancer. I was in. I wanted to be a part of that team. I was going to help eliminate childhood cancer!

As fate would have it, I applied to an externship to learn more about their approach to cancer when I was in nursing school. After filling out a paper application, passing a phone interview, and then flying to Memphis for an in-person interview, I was SHOCKED to find out that I was one of four nursing students chosen from a pool of 4800 students to extern at St. Jude's Children's Research Hospital for an entire summer. It was a dream come true. Now, this wasn't required by my school. I chose this. In fact, my hope was to earn a job offer and stay at St. Jude's. I remember arriving at the hospital and fan-girling so hard that I was at the hospital that you see in all the commercials. The place I had fundraised for, for so long.

That summer was intense and would shape my heart for cancer in ways that I wouldn't be able to really work on till nearly a decade later.

The place that I really thought would do the research to eradicate childhood cancer as we know it. And I would be a part of the team that could help that mission! That summer was intense and would shape my heart for cancer in ways that I wouldn't be able to really work on till nearly a decade later. I remember hanging bags of meds for kids and wondering if they were getting some life-saving drug this family was praying for or if it was simply saline. As part of a double-blind placebo test, none of us knew. The reality of what it was to be in a clinical trial, was crazy to me. As a last-ditch effort, some of the toughest cases in the world would come there, to further research and find a cure. Yet a cure was never guaranteed.

That summer was filled with playing hide and seek on the floor with kids, talking to teens in their last days, comforting families as they put on brave faces, and simply trying to make life as normal as possible even while we were all acutely aware of the reality of the situation. We'd play tooth fairy when a child would lose a tooth. They'd throw proms for kids that couldn't make it to theirs. We'd have celebrities come visit for "Make a Wish." It seemed like such a magical place.

I remember one girl that would bring a shoebox that would collect her braids as they would fall out each time she was inpatient for chemo, and would laugh about which color wig she would chose this time, and loved being the "diva." These kids were here for clinical trials of experimental drugs. For many, this was their last hope. If St. Jude's couldn't do it, there was nothing left to be done. In my heart, I couldn't bear not doing whatever it took to help these kids.

At the end of that summer, I was offered not one but two positions! This was truly an answer to prayer, but it wasn't the only answered prayer. Remember that dream about Simon? I discovered I was pregnant with him at the same time I was at St. Jude! The children there had stolen my heart forever, and one of them even inspired my son's middle name. However, our growing family was just the thing to bring us back to Wisconsin, where I ultimately wanted to be closer to family while raising mine.

Okay, so let's put it all together. I am a nurse, and I have a heart for cancer patients; my own health restoration journey from autoimmune conditions and fertility challenges brought me to The Wellness Way…and now 2020 seems to be the catalyst for what appears to be the perfect storm for a huge influx of autoimmune conditions and cancer that would soon flood the office. And just like that, I'm back in my sweet spot, giving people more options and hope than I ever could have in medical practice.

In November of 2022, I was working with a team to officially launch The Wellness Way's Metabolic Approach to Cancer program in January 2023. The need became so great that I couldn't wait. Like, really, couldn't wait. I had patients coming in, ready or not! I was seeing patients before we could even get the clinic fully prepared! Our clinic reception area became a makeshift IV room during off hours. We were often making materials on the fly to support the patients starting this new program. We were in such high demand we couldn't hold back. In fact, at this point, we have a waiting list. We are training more practitioners to be able to help support this important need. But why? What is The Wellness Way doing to support cancer patients that is so different from the other options they have?

Let's talk a little bit about cancer, then we can dive into that. Ready for some scary stats? One out of two men and one out of 2.4 women will receive a cancer diagnosis in their lifetime. Look around you. Who do you know who has cancer? Most people have a cancering process going on 8-10 years before it is diagnosed. And many of those diagnosis come from screening techniques, they're not even aware of it before that. People go in for mammograms or a colonoscopy and they

Did you know that up to 95% of cancers are preventable and are due to lifestyle?

happen to find it. But did you know that up to 95% of cancers are preventable and are due to lifestyle? Only about 5% are due to damaged DNA!

I know those stats all sound very grim and not really encouraging, but there is hope! Stick with me! Cancer is NOT a tumor. Cancer is a process. The tumor is merely a symptom of a sick body. We all have cells that could potentially form a cancer at any given time, when there's enough "chinks in the armor" so-to-speak. By looking at how the body functions as a whole, we can identify those "chinks" to strengthen the armor against disease. Such "chinks" could include things like blood sugar imbalances, mental stress, imbalanced circadian rhythm, high toxic burden, hormonal imbalances, immune system dysfunction, issues with the microbiome etc. If you are aware of how your body is functioning, you can help support it so that it can either handle the cancer cells or help so that your body can eliminate the harmful cells before they can take root. It's possible, and we are doing it every day!

SOMATIC VS. METABOLIC APPROACH TO CANCER

In the world of cancer, there are two main approaches. The somatic and the metabolic theories lay out two very different explanations and strategies as to why cancer exists and how to fight it.

Many people are most aware of the somatic approach. Tell me if this sounds familiar: The tumor is evil, and the cells have to be eradicated at any and all cost to the body! Cancer is due to crappy genes and is basically a terrible game of Russian Roulette. You have no power in this. And, once therapy starts, eat whatever you want, just don't lose weight! With a 70% reoccurrence rate, how's that working for us? We are addressing the tumor only – the symptom - and not asking 'what are the risk factors that led to the formation of that tumor in the first place?' Each individual is subject to a protocol based on their tumor type. However, if there are five patients with the

> **Cancer is NOT a tumor. Cancer is a process.**

same diagnosis, they may have similar patterns in their history, but ultimately, they have five very individual chronologies that led to that diagnosis. Do you think they should all be treated the same?

Let me give you a little insight. Standard of Care evaluates reoccurrence rates at 5 years because looking out any further would expose the lack of success. We have been fighting the "war on cancer" since 1971 when Richard Nixon signed the National Cancer Act and have spent billions of dollars researching the human genome, genetic links to cancer, and yet we are no further along in finding a cure than we were back then. Clearly, this approach is lackluster at best.

Then there's the metabolic theory which believes that your tumor may have actually saved your life. Hang with me here. The body is very intelligent in everything that it does. So if you have abnormal cells going helter-skelter throughout the body, you would have died a long time ago! Your body took all of those abnormal cells and put them in one spot, which ends up being the tumor so that they're not running rampant all throughout your body. By keeping it all contained, your body very intelligently says, all right, now I have something that I can fight! It gives the body one target to focus on. It's what is keeping you alive without allowing the toxins to spill over. Blood cancers obviously behave differently, as many outside influences such as toxins, viruses and sugar make the blood itself sick. But the blood didn't make a mistake when it became sick – it was simply responding to its environment.

The metabolic approach also looks at which fuels cancers prefer. Think about it this way. Cancer LOVES sugar. Like a lot.

Cancer LOVES sugar. Like a lot. If we know that, we can set up the battleground to win!

If we know that, we can set up the battleground to win! How is your body metabolizing sugars? How is your insulin reacting? What type of personalized eating plan would be most therapeutic for you? There are many drivers in the cancer story...sugar is just one of them. Other drivers can include toxins, mental traumas, viruses, bacteria, fungi, inflammatory triggers, hormones that are not metabolized properly, etc. When we have proper testing, we can determine the answers to those questions, what is driving your particular cancer and get you started on the right path!

Remember earlier when I said up to 95% of cancers are preventable and due to lifestyle, and only about 5% are due to damaged DNA? Most cancer begins before DNA damage. Mitochondria are the genome protector and need the right fuel sources and protection from the 3Ts (Dr. Patrick talked about that

192

awhile back in the book!). The signals, based on the nourishment they receive, tell the cells how to function and replicate. When those mitochondria and cells can't die properly (remember, that's good! Your body has to renew its cells continuously!) and take the "trash" out, everything becomes mucky. What comes from that muck? Illness, unhealthy, abnormal cells. Cancer. We have to support the mitochondria and be able to break down and kill off the rogue cells! Mitochondria are the good guys! You want lots of good healthy ones!

Let's explain it this way. One of my favorite analogies that I have seen taught and communicated over and over is the fishbowl analogy. If a fish is swimming around in murky water, over time that fish will become sick. You can remove the fish from the tank and "treat" the fish by cutting out sick organs, poisoning the fish, and removing anything from the fish's body that is the evidence of the sickness, and make it good as new. But if that fish is then placed back into the murky water, it is only a matter of time before that fish will become sick again. And now that the fish has some residual damage, or is missing pieces and parts from the first time it was fixed, it will be harder to fight the second time. This is the reason why we can be so good at getting the person into remission, but when it comes back, we're not as good at "fixing" it the second time. The cancer becomes more aggressive and more resistant to treatment. Eventually we push the body past it's limits and we kill the person faster than we kill the tumor. Cleaning the tank takes time, and effort, and lifelong changes in behavior. But it is possible to have healing, if you can figure out what is making the water murky in the first place.

Adipose (fat) tissue has less mitochondrial activity. Muscle tissue has way more! You need to keep your body fat content in mind. Fat is a great hiding ground for those toxins! So, body fat is something you can reduce so that your toxin load can be reduced, and your body can more efficiently eliminate those harmful substances! Just know that if you start on a journey to lose weight and you have a heavy toxin load, it is a good idea to connect with a doctor or practitioner who can guide you through so that you can effectively eliminate those toxins instead of simply having them circulate and cause more challenges.

Maybe you or a family member with cancer has been told you can do chemotherapy or radiation or hormonal therapy, and it's either that or nothing. Maybe you've been told there is nothing else to be done. You've exhausted all of your options. First of all, I disagree! And I'm here to tell you today that there are a lot of options. And we have time. We have time to pause and evaluate with comprehensive testing and a detailed plan.

NOT A ONE OR THE OTHER, BUT A BEAUTIFUL "AND"

Okay, let's be honest. If you've read this far, you are totally aware of how The Wellness Way must be seen from the perspective of the medical community. I'll give you a hint, we aren't loved, and patients aren't encouraged to come see us by their doctors. In fact, many times, my patients feel the need to go rogue and see me underground. That makes for some interesting testing discussions...

Many people assume this means that other Wellness Way practitioners and I would not support a patient seeing an oncologist for chemo or radiation. That's not entirely true!

Oncologists are the experts on the tumor and how to destroy it. I focus on the terrain, and how to support the body through treatment.

Remember the Fireman and Carpenter analogy? It is important to know which professional to call in which situation. Cancer is not a single disease with just one approach. Each person developed cancer for a specific reason. And each person will need a personalized approach to help support their body to eliminate those cells.

If we take the time to do the proper testing, we can do just that. I oftentimes tell people that oncologists are the experts on the tumor and how to destroy the tumor. I focus on the terrain, and how to support the body through treatment.

Another point I wish to make and take home is that cancer is rarely an emergency. Many people have been fighting cancer without even knowing it for 8-10 years before there is ever a diagnosis. Most of the time we don't need to rush into decisions on surgery, radiation, or chemotherapy the next day. We have time to evaluate and test the body to make sure that the plan they have laid out is the best plan for them, and that their body is strong enough to tolerate it. I always tell my patients that I want them to make decisions for them based on data, not based on fear. And that if they can give me a couple weeks to collect the data and go over the pros and cons of every decision before starting treatment, that they will not regret it. They will have better results when we can support the body through treatment and give it what it needs.

Listen to me closely. I am not against the standard of care. And for the majority of patients, it's not going to be an either-or, but a very beautiful and where we can use different weapons that we have within the standard of care alongside optimizing your immune response, working on your microbiome, working on your body so that standard of care options can work better. Our goal as a team is to make their treatments more effective and less toxic, so you can tolerate treatment longer and get the result. Our goal is to simultaneously help the body in it's fight against the cancer while also addressing the terrain that developed the cancer in the first place.

There are four *Ps* that make up our strategy. When we have proper testing, each month we evaluate if what we are doing is working. We take these labs to help us make calls on knowing when we need to *PUSH* the body harder, when we need to *PAUSE*, when we may just need to *PULL BACK* a minute, or if it's time to *PIVOT* our plan completely. If we're on round five of chemotherapy and things are going great, we keep on going. If we look at the immune system and we look at some of those different terrain labs, and it shows that your body is falling apart, maybe we pause. And that's okay, we can pause, we can pivot, we can change direction at any step. People believe the fallacy that if they pause treatment their cancer will suddenly grow out of control. But that's not the case. If the body isn't stable and there isn't anywhere for that treatment to land, then it will be an ineffective treatment. We never want to get into a situation in which we are killing the patient faster than we are killing the tumor.

What if the best choice for you is surgery? We need to prepare the body and listen to what it needs. It's always giving clues. What if there are certain things that we can give your body in advance of the surgery for better outcomes and recovery? Did you know there are certain times of a menstrual cycle that lead to better outcomes for a lumpectomy or mastectomy? This is why that detailed strategy is more important than simply taking the first available time on an OR calendar.

What if your insulin or blood sugar is too high as you are preparing for radiation? You may be doing a whole lot more harm than good. In fact, radiation without taking some key factors into consideration can lead to more aggressive and rogue cells. If you go into radiation with high sugar, high insulin, and high VEGF, that radiation treatment is actually contraindicated as it will make some stem cells stronger and more resistant to treatment later on. These are things we can test ahead of time to see if your body is ready and prepared for the best outcomes from radiation. But, with complete testing and looking at cancer from a metabolic approach, you can set the body up to be prepared for the radiation to do as the doctor explained it could do. Ever wonder why when two people with the same exact cancer, same exact treatment, same exact dose, same exact protocol that could have vastly different outcomes? If treatment works independent of the terrain in which those treatments land, they would work 100% of the time. Yet we aren't seeing that. Each individual going through treatment has different starting points for their health, and THAT is what makes the difference in their outcome. NOT the protocol that was chosen for them.

How is your mitochondrial health? In Standard of Care, we destroy the tumor and any circulating cancer cells with chemotherapy and radiation. But that destruction of the cancer cells is not targeting just the cancer – it destroys healthy cells too. It's what it does! But what if you could prepare your body to protect the healthy cells as much as possible so they can help "take out the trash" that the chemo creates? Consider this -- what if you left trash piled up in your house for a week? What would happen? It would get putrid! Mitochondria is the powerhouse of the cell and is what makes that cell healthy, and provides the body with energy. Are you fatigued? That is the number one sign of mitochondrial insufficiency. Since the mitochondria makes energy, if they aren't working properly it results in fatigue. Mitochondria are influenced by the external environment. Set these powerhouses up for success by taking care of them and waging war with them, not against them! They are the key players in forming a metabolic approach to cancer.

Need more convincing that this all has to do with the terrain and not necessarily the genetic expression of a tumor? Let's take the nuclei transfer cell studies as an example. The nucleus of the cell is what contains all the genetic information for that particular cell. So if the nucleus of the cell contained altered DNA, then the theory would be that it would present as a cancer cell. So to prove this point, what they did was take the nucleus of a cancer cell, and insert it into a healthy cell. They thought that this would turn the healthy cell into a cancer cell, but much to their surprise it did not. The opposite was also true. They took the nucleus of a healthy cell and put inside a healthy cell and thought it would make that cell healthy. But it did not. If cancer was strictly a genetic disease, then they should create more cancer by injecting it with that genetic blueprint, correct? What they discovered through these studies is that it is not the DNA or the nucleus that determines the nature of that cell, but rather the mitochondria – that is sick or healthy in response to the environment in which it resides.

What you need is someone that can ask the right questions about what created the cancer in the first place. When you have the answers to all the questions, the results of all the tests, and a different perspective, you will be equipped to make decisions from a place of confidence instead of fear. That, my friend, makes all the difference.

TERRAIN CONCEPT

I've done extensive education in integrative oncology and the metabolic approach to cancer as inspired by the work of Dr. Thomas Seyfried, and mentored by those in the field who have brought that research into practice such as Dr. Nasha Winters. I have also been trained in mistletoe therapies and anthroposophic medicine. Through all of these studies I have found that although cancer is never, never a blessing, it is an opportunity to pause and take inventory of your life as we know it, from your health to your relationships to everything else in between.

Many times people say, "Gosh, I was very healthy until I had cancer." That just simply cannot be the case. I would argue that most people have a cancering process happening in their body for 8-10 years before there ever is an abnormality that shows up in a lab or on a scan. This cancer is something that's probably been brewing in your life for a really long time with risk factors that you may have never considered addressing.

Remember when I mentioned 90% to 95% of cancer diagnoses have come about because of poor diets, poor lifestyle changes, and other things that we're exposed to?

Think of this analogy. We're all born with a bucket. Then we encounter mental stress, and we have toxic burden, and we have microbiome dysfunction, and we have medications, and we have environmental exposures.

Eventually, that bucket is going to overflow. I'm here to help you take inventory of that bucket and try to figure out what is all in that bucket. How do we start to reverse engineer all the life exposure that filled your bucket to be able to give you the healthiest body that you've ever had before?

At The Wellness Way, what we do is start to digest all of that. We go deep into who you are, your physiological biography, so to speak. I care about where your parents grew up. I care about if you were born naturally or via C-section. I care about whether you were breastfed or bottle-fed.

> **We have to take inventory of what that environment is doing within your body.**

I care about the environment in which you grew up and the different toxic exposures that you've had from a very young age, a lot of things that were beyond your control. I care about your family history. I care about all of those details. And so, working with the metabolic approach to cancer, we come at it from the perspective of the fact that your body is not broken. It is simply adapting to the environment it is in and each of the 3Ts it faces daily.

Every single one of us has stem cells that could turn into cancer at any moment. So, what is the difference between someone whose stem cells do turn to cancer and someone whose doesn't? It has everything to do with the environment. I love to say, "Genetics loads the gun, but lifestyle and the environment pull the trigger."

We have to take inventory of what that environment is doing within your body. So we look at things like your microbiome, we look at your hormones, we look at food allergies. We look at what your immune system is doing.

We look at your blood sugar balance. We look at your mental health scores.

We look at your adverse childhood event scores. We look up your zip code and find out what environmental toxins/exposures you have. We look up what toxins may be found in your drinking water. We take all that data and lay it out in front of us to determine the right course of action for you. Many times, people think that they have to choose between Western medicine and a more natural approach or The Wellness Way Approach.

I want to be very, very clear here. The Wellness Way does not treat cancer. I'm not going to come up with a natural treatment plan for you to go through. What we do instead is create an environment in the body that is inhospitable to cancer. We starve those cancer cells of sugar, which has been proven time and time again as a fuel source for those cancer cells. We help to address the hormones that might be feeding a tumoring process. We work on restoring the microbiome and ensuring those detox pathways are prepared so your body can get rid of toxins that may have built up in your system over time.

When you look at the body as a host, as a healthy, not broken, intelligent and functional entity, you can take back control of your health, even in the midst of battling cancer. Just like any war, the right strategy makes all the difference!

Well meaning "natural" doctors can do the same thing as traditional medical providers if they are not careful. They tend to react out of fear, instead of strategy, and implement protocols instead of personalized medicine, which is why this approach only works for a handful of people as well. Many times in my practice I have seen the right therapy applied at the wrong time and it creates poor outcomes. Even interventions such as high dose Vitamin C, hyperbaric oxygen and ozone have incredible utility. But the right therapy applied at the wrong time is the wrong therapy. This is where we need to be keeping close tabs on your labs, know which therapy is appropriate at the right times, to get you the best results.

THERE'S HOPE! YOUR BODY WANTS TO HEAL!

We have so many fantastic stories coming out of our clinic daily. I could tell you about parents who were told there was nothing they could do, the doctors felt they didn't even have anything to offer, who are now celebrating life with their kids. Cancer free!

I could tell you about people who were ready to give up, but then looked at their family and realized they had to continue the fight. And now, they are planning a life with those families!

I could tell you about children coming in, that had the childhood cancer that I wanted to be a part of eradicating. Today, I know that what I am offering them, the bags our team hangs, is filled with the lifesaving compounds their bodies need. There is a vibrant hope for these youngsters in the dawn of their lives! Here is a patient Dr. Patrick supported through a cancering process. The Wellness Way has been able to help and support cancer patients since before I started this program.

NATALIE'S STORY

Since 2016 I have had roughly 45 radiation treatments, 42 immunotherapy treatments, four biopsies, four different cancer medications, months of constant vomiting, countless tears, hours in prayer, and numerous doctors telling me there was no possibility for a cure or any healing. Still, I refused to give up.

The renal cell carcinoma I had in 2010 had come back, this time in my bone. Over the summer of 2016, I completed several radiation treatments and took an oral chemo medication. I did so well on that treatment that my oncologist recommended I no longer take it due to the severity of the drug and the dormancy of my cancer cells. Well, fast forward to 2019; the cancer became so catastrophic that I lost the ability to walk. My left hip socket was all but gone, my femur and pelvis fractured, and the pain was nearly unbearable. Because of this, I have been on crutches for almost three years. Stage 4 renal cell carcinoma.

No cure. No healing. The goal was to slow its growth to buy me more time. That was the best they could hope for, per the oncologists.

It was terrifying, and we felt like we were in no man's land. But we were never alone.

During the hardest moments, God would outweigh my disparity with hope and encouragement. Sometimes, it was an encouraging sermon. Other times, a surprise delivery of flowers or gift baskets. There were times I came home and found our front porch plastered with encouraging Bible verses, books, gifts, and food. Hundreds and hundreds of people rallied around Blake and me in prayer: family, friends, and total strangers. Fundraisers were held in my honor, and prayer circles were hosted across many cities and states. I received enough handwritten notes and cards to fill a Hallmark store. As time went on, I would bounce back after each devastating scan report I would receive. There were moments when I felt like I was taking steps backward. It seemed my health was going in the opposite direction. I wouldn't take it to heart when I heard, "We may have to explore other options if your next scan shows more growth."

I first learned about The Wellness Way from my best friend. She was working with a doctor from the network who was helping her with her hormones. She encouraged me for months to schedule an appointment. I was convinced my constant juicing and raw diet were the answers to my healing, so I didn't take the time.

In 2020, when my health was deteriorating again, and I was on crutches, I started watching Dr. Flynn's videos. I would watch and take notes on every single video or live message. One day on his show, he spoke about a young woman he had helped with an inoperable brain tumor and then had her share her story. She was thriving, and her tumor was gone or almost undetectable! I remember the tears in my eyes, wondering if Dr. Flynn could help me.

I immediately reached out and called his office. When I was told that he wasn't accepting new patients, I was so disappointed and left it alone. I remember praying and asking God that if Dr. Flynn were supposed to be a part of my care, He would make it happen. Well, fast forward to the spring of 2020; that same best friend knew Erika Downs, a soon-to-be graduating doctor from chiropractor school. Erika was personal friends with Dr. Flynn and trained under him. My best friend shared my story with Erika and told me that Erika had promised to talk to Dr. Flynn. Again, I prayed that if Dr. Flynn were supposed to be a part of my care, God would make it happen. Sure enough, Dr. Erika Downs reached out to me and gathered my story to present to Dr. Flynn. Dr. Flynn then called me and asked to hear my story personally. Then he told me about the plan he was putting together. The Wellness Way doctors are so thorough! They began by requesting blood work with specific markers in mind. I had never had testing like this in all the years of treating the cancer ravaging my body.

My labs were terrible. I remember Dr. Patrick calling me to say my immune system was like a sports team with no coach. He took the time to explain each test and why cancer was taking over my body. Dr. Erika Downs, who was also seeing me here locally in my hometown, told me Dr. Flynn had called her to share his thoughts and consult with her. I trusted them because no specialist had ever looked at my bloodwork to see the big picture.

I started a series of supplements and restrictive eating. The cancer was fast and aggressive, and Dr. Flynn encouraged me to do combination therapy. I was so grateful for him because he was the only clinician who told me healing could happen. He explained that it took a long time for my body to get this way, and it would take time to heal. Before starting the supplements, my labs and numbers were so depleted I was a couple of points away from needing a blood transfusion. Within a couple of weeks, my labs started to trend up! It was so reassuring to me to see the results and know that I was making the right decision.

Dr. Flynn is so real and genuine. He was constantly checking to see if I needed anything. Whenever he shared his knowledge and insights, it always checked out with my own research. Dr. Flynn is constantly studying and adding to his knowledge. He keeps learning to support his patients with the best care possible. His commitment to continuing education built so much confidence and helped reassure me that I was in the right place. He encouraged me in a very dark time of my life. I will forever be grateful for his hope and positivity.

Dr. Erika Downs was an angel and so helpful and encouraging. She would read medical textbooks just to better assist me. Dr. Flynn would reach out to Dr. Erika to see how I was doing, and she would reach out to him to keep him updated. I truly had a dynamic team!

Dr. Flynn visited my hometown area to do one of his life-changing talks. When Dr. Erika introduced us, I cried as I hugged him. I was so excited to meet him and for all he had done for me. I knew I would forever be beyond grateful to him. He is such a wealth of knowledge with a huge heart.

From the beginning, l always felt I would be healed. I had received peace that cancer would not be my end. The Lord gave me so much hope and joy. I knew healing was coming, and so did my prayer warriors. Today, I can proudly proclaim that I have received news that not only are the cancer cells in my body dying off, but my bones have miraculously REGROWN. They have healed to the point that I can walk without assistance. No more crutches. No more wheelchair. The moment Blake and I so desperately waited and prayed for is here. The impossible has happened. We cannot begin to describe the whirlwind of emotions over this life-changing miracle.

I needed both the firemen and the carpenters; both teams have been so necessary in this journey!

Thank you to the doctors at the Wellness Way who provided so much guidance and teaching and were always cheering me on! Thank you! I needed both the firemen and the carpenters; both teams have been so necessary in this journey!

But I give the most thanks to God above. I was not curable. My bones were destroyed. Because of God, I stand today as a literal WALKING miracle. My life has defied all the odds. Our joy cannot be contained or described in words.

Who's up for a 5k?

WHAT CAN YOU DO TODAY?

Nobody likes to talk about cancer and especially not their own mortality. I want you to know cancer isn't some game of Russian Roulette where you have no power. In fact, you have more power than you know! You just have to know what that is, and how to use it. Our doctors help patients with this every day. Not just to avoid a cancer diagnosis but to restore proper function and health.

Are you ready for the secret? Actually, it's not really a secret, but if it caused you to sit up a little straighter and take notes, good! Cancer can't occur in a healthy body. I know you may not have been born into a perfect world. This isn't Eden, my friend. But there are things you can do to help support your body and restore that function.

Think back to that bucket. There are ten streams that can add drops to cause your bucket to overflow. If you optimize the bucket, you optimize your health! What are they? Dr. Nasha Winters refers to these 10 areas of the terrain as the Terrain 10, and if any number of these areas are off, disease can present.

Your gut microbiome. How is everything flowing? Is what's going in actually being used as nutrients by the body and waste being taken out? Properly, and effectively? Are you able to absorb, convert, and break down nutrients as your body is designed to? Is the good flora in the right balance? Heck, do you have more good flora than bad? Are there any parasites?

Genetic and epigenetic history. Okay, let me set this straight. Your body is designed for health. But you may have some physiological history from your family tree that doesn't look good. Do you know that you can support those "bad genes" so they don't express themselves? Your body isn't broken! It may just need a little bit more TLC in some areas.

Blood sugar balance. Ugh, I know, I know...Doc already hit on this. Nobody craves a salad, everyone craves the sugar. Well, if you've come this far, you also know that cancer does, too! Your body has to be flexible enough to handle the fuel sources it needs to run. And you have to provide it the right ones for proper function!

Circulation and angiogenesis. How's your blood flowing? Do you have issues with the way that your heart is pumping? Are you on blood pressure medication? Are those nutrients able to make it to where they should once your gut and other organs have set the stage? Circulation isn't simply a heart concern, it's literally the highway of your body to deliver nutrients!

Hormone balance. You just read it from the main man. Read the first half of the book again if you need to!

Toxic burden. What are you exposed to daily? What "foods" that aren't really nourishing foods are you taking in? What are you rubbing onto your skin? Ladies, what are you reapplying on the daily? Fellas, what chemicals are you working in and around? And...that perfect lawn? Likely toxic! Toxins are everywhere and we can't avoid them all, but if you avoid what you can, you'll reduce your overall load!

Inflammation. This is a biggie. Inflammation is a big red sign from your body. Quite literally. Inflammation can be anywhere, including internal. One of the biggest things I recommend is taking a look at your food allergies. Often this is a source of hidden inflammation most people ignore.

Immune function. Doc just laid this out in a previous chapter. Immune function is critical to keeping you alive from foreign proteins and managing inflammation. Hint, vaccines and drugs don't support healthy immune function!

Now, the two nobody wants to hear about. If you thought we got push back from the food and favorite product side, buckle up!

Mental stress. Yep, there it is again! Doc said it earlier, it is one of the biggest contributor to illness for women. In the past several years, it's only increased across the board with no signs of decreasing. Don't tell me you can't reduce it. I know life continues on. You have to find a way to manage it so that it doesn't affect your overall health.

Circadian rhythm. Go to bed!!! Seriously! It is that simple. Think about the rhythm of the sun and how our ancestors used to structure their days. You need good, restorative, replenishing sleep, and that takes good sleep hygiene. Do you need to unplug the wifi? Do you need to lay out your clothes before you go to bed so you can get up and out of the house on time? Maybe put the kids to bed earlier? Set some boundaries with some teens? Throw the phone in a drawer? Men, get about 7-8 hours per night. And help your ladies get the 8-10 they need. That's right, she *needs* it.

When you understand who you are, your strengths and weaknesses, and how to best support your body, you can make the best choices. This doesn't just apply to a cancer treatment plan, but how to avoid one!

I want to close with two things. I hope I never see you in our cancer care clinic. But, if you ever need us, you know where to find us. We are The Wellness Way. And we are here to help.

CHAPTER 16

CHOLESTEROL IS NOT A BAD GUY.

"My doctor says my hormones are so low I should be on these synthetic hormones," a woman tells me after a recent seminar. It's not the first time. In fact, I hear it often. So, I ask her, "Are you taking a statin or cholesterol altering medication?" She said, "yes." I'm going to tell you what I told her, the several other women that came up to me that day with the same statement, and what I told the thousands of other women throughout the years: If you are taking a statin drug you can never achieve hormonal balance. Women aren't the only ones. Men are being told they need to take statins, too. This is one of the biggest struggles in medicine, especially as the rate of people on statins is skyrocketing.

Over 25% of American adults over the age of forty have taken a statin drug in the past thirty days. From 2009-2019 there was a 197% increase in statin drug prescriptions. Will statins lower your cholesterol? Yes. But let's start this conversation by first understanding cholesterol and how it got the reputation it has.

Cholesterol got a bad reputation a long time ago because it was assumed it had a role in arterial plaque formation; that idea still continues through traditional medical thinking. Cholesterol was, and still is, found in high numbers at the site of arterial plaquing. Many people thought that because it was there, it was the cause of the plaque formation which would eventually build up and lead to a heart attack.

Your body makes roughly 2,000 – 3,000 milligrams of cholesterol a day. Diet change can only impact our cholesterol level by maybe 10%. Lots of you gave up eggs, shrimp, and other healthy foods to have an impact on your cholesterol levels, and ultimately you were given statin drugs to lower your cholesterol—cholesterol your body needs.

We need to look deeper though, especially with all we are learning in our thinking. It's easy to blame cholesterol but remember how the body works and that it doesn't make mistakes. We need to understand what cholesterol does, and how it works with male and female hormones. This is going to be fun—something I bet you've never heard of before!

Okay, a quick recap, if you will. We have talked about how hormones are messengers. That's what they do. Steroid hormones are a group of chemical messaging compounds produced by male and female sex organs, the adrenal glands, and the kidneys (mineralocorticoid). It's your testosterone, your estrogens, your progesterone, and other important hormones that keep your body functioning. We got that. Hormones are important and interconnected to your whole body. Hormones involve multiple organs. A lot of steroid hormones are produced in one organ but then go to another and are converted in that organ for function. We will learn a little more about that later in the steroid pathway chart. It will be important to remember that every organ needs messages. There are lots of hormones bringing messages throughout your body helping it function. Steroid hormones impact a lot of your body's functions like blood pressure, bone density, and your kidneys. It's not just about male and female cycle differences. Got that? Okay, let's go on.

If the message is messed up there are going to be hormonal imbalances. For example, take a hormone like estradiol. If the message delivered is too high it can possibly develop into cancer, or too low may lead to depression or early menopause. The tissue will listen if it gets the message, but it doesn't mean it's the right message for that individual. All of our organs are controlled by messengers and the messengers can affect multiple organs. Medicine in its classification separates everything. We have heart specialists, brain specialists, kidney specialists, GI specialists. We need those specialists, but the trouble we run into is they limit their scope to one organ. We need to realize messengers can affect all those organs, not just the one the specialist is focused on.

You can see how important hormones are to the overall balance of the body or homeostasis. Guess where they come from. Are you ready? The building blocks of steroid hormones (and a lot of other important cells) is cholesterol. Your body needs cholesterol, along with luteinizing hormone, to make steroid hormones. All steroid hormones are derived from cholesterol. Let's be clear—not all hormones, but all steroid hormones. Which ones are those? Sex hormones, adrenal hormones, and kidney hormones. They all need cholesterol.

As you can see in the chart below, all these hormones start as cholesterol, and then become the hormones needed for a wide variety of functions. Cholesterol is a derivative. It's not bad for you. It's a building block for every steroid hormone in the body. You don't want a goal of no cholesterol. If you do, you will affect your hormones. Zero cholesterol means zero hormones. And that's a bad day!

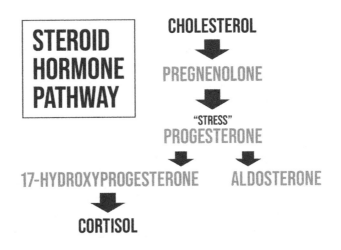

Why is your cholesterol high? That is the magic question. Your body will make cholesterol when you're under stress. It actually needs cholesterol to repair itself or when it needs more hormones. If I cut my finger and start bleeding, then my body is going to make more cholesterol to repair the wound.

Cholesterol isn't the bad guy here; cholesterol is the police.

When medical thinking saw the cholesterol at the site of plaque formation, they incorrectly blamed the cholesterol. Just because the police are at the scene of a crime doesn't mean they are the ones that caused the crime. Whenever there is damage or inflammation, cholesterol has to go there to protect and heal the area. Cholesterol isn't the bad guy here; cholesterol is the police. Cholesterol is doing its job to heal and protect. The body is doing its job when it sends the cholesterol to the site that needs help and support. This misconception leads to the frequent prescription of cholesterol lowering medications. Cholesterol is needed all over and travels via the bloodstream to every single part of the body.

Let's put the pieces together. If you are a woman and your adrenals get fatigued because of stress as hormones get low, your cholesterol will go up. It's your body responding by creating what it needs to adapt to what is going on and heal itself. It's not because cholesterol is this bad guy that is intruding in your body. It's not because you are eating too much cholesterol.

If your cholesterol goes up, there is a physical reason why. 80+% is made by the liver.

Your body makes roughly 2,000 – 3,000 milligrams of cholesterol a day. Diet change can only impact our cholesterol level by maybe 10%. Lots of you gave up eggs, shrimp, and other healthy foods to have an impact on your cholesterol levels, and ultimately you were given statin drugs to lower your cholesterol—cholesterol your body needs.

Think about it—the body does not make mistakes. Your liver makes the majority of cholesterol in your body. Do you suppose the liver would actually make something that's bad for the heart? Knowing what you now know, does that even make sense? Multiple studies have shown that dietary cholesterol does not increase coronary artery disease. Researchers are calling for guidelines to be reconsidered but unfortunately many people are still being treated under this outdated and disproven perspective. Cholesterol is typically high because the body is under stress or there is some major hormonal deficiency.

When I see high LDL on a guy's lab, and he has low testosterone, I know what the body is doing. The body says low testosterone? What do I need to make more? Cholesterol. I will be thrilled when we all understand how this works!

The question is: what stress, inflammation, or hormonal deficiency is causing your body to create more cholesterol? I'm not going to drop it down with red yeast rice or statin drugs. I'm going to look into why it is high. It can be different based on the individual and very different based on sex. Anyone with chronic inflammation, stress, hormonal imbalances, autoimmune issues, leaky gut, and many other health issues all NEED higher cholesterol levels to heal. The idea of creating an average or even an ideal level for cholesterol baffles me because levels can and should change dramatically when someone has some of those health issues.

Cholesterol is the building block for all tissues and hormones in the body and is not a bad thing. High cholesterol is a sign that something in the body isn't functioning properly, and more cholesterol is needed to heal. Artificially lowering cholesterol with statin medication interferes with this healing process and makes people sicker.

Cholesterol has many roles beyond hormones that we can be affecting if we are prescribing medications to lower it. Just by looking at a few of those roles we can see how critical cholesterol is to our Swiss watch.

Cell membranes rely heavily on cholesterol. Every cell in our body is surrounded by a cell membrane. Cholesterol gives the cell membrane flexibility in addition to the strength and support necessary to maintain its shape.

We need cholesterol for optimal nerve, brain, and memory function. Our nerve cells are specialized cells that transmit information throughout the body. Cholesterol allows for faster and higher quality transmission of those signals. What part of the body has the highest cholesterol? The highest amount of cholesterol is found in the brain. The brain relies on cholesterol for overall function, specifically for memory formation and retention. You can see why cholesterol becomes even more important as we age, and we have a higher demand on our brain functions. Yet, which age range is almost always on a statin? Our elderly! This is crazy!

Cholesterol is a precursor for vitamin D production that is synthesized in the skin. Vitamin D is vital for your immunity along with your physical and mental well-being.

Gallbladder function is heavily reliant on the help of cholesterol. Cholesterol is converted into bile salts allowing the digestive process to emulsify fats properly. Gallbladder surgeries are on the rise! I wonder how many gallbladder surgeries could be prevented if cholesterol levels supported normal bile salt production?

High cholesterol is a sign that something in the body isn't functioning properly and more cholesterol is needed to heal.

This is just scratching the surface of the importance of cholesterol and why we need it. I understand this is a big shift in understanding, and some of you may still fear cholesterol. Don't govern your health care choices by fear! The drugs work on cholesterol, but the picture is so much bigger! More and more people are suffering the side effects of the drugs. It says right on the product insert in the prescription box that the side effects are low hormones, renal disease, depression, impotence, and more. I see these effects in patients in my office every day. I disagree that people have to live a life on these drugs, suffering the side effects. There is a different way to do healthcare.

Statins are shown to affect the heart. Statins interfere with the production of LDL which interfere with CoQ10. What organ does CoQ10 fuel? Your heart. Wait! Hold the phone! Why would you take a drug for your heart that can have a bad effect on the heart? This just doesn't make sense!

Studies show that statins lower testosterone. If you lower cholesterol, you lower testosterone which increases rates of impotence. So, statins can cause drug induced impotence. Don't worry, the drug company that makes one of the top-selling statins, Lipitor, also makes Viagra. You may have heard of them: Pfizer. If a guy is taking a statin drug and his testosterone goes down, what are some of the side effects of the medication? Impotence, heart disease (the very thing it is supposed to help with), loss of motivation, weight gain. That's all on the drug packet insert. Then, we have male enhancement drugs. Let's think about that. They created the problem with one drug. Now they've created another drug to solve the problem created by the first drug. That's what they know to do, but it's not going to bring the results most people want. How many prescriptions do you need to be healthy? That's big money-making in the billions. Even though it seems like common sense, we can see in studies and anecdotal evidence that lowering cholesterol negatively impacts steroid hormones.

You can maintain a normal hormone balance from the day you were born until the day you die.

Remember how often I hear this one? "My doctor says my hormones are low because of my age." For them, the hormones may be low because they are on statins. When they get tested and follow their personalized course of care with a

Wellness Way doctor, they find they may be able to get off statin drugs and synthetic hormones and maintain proper hormonal balance and ranges. That's when I say to them, "Good thing you got younger, your hormones are balanced!" They look at me like I'm nuts and let me know they are actually older. They are indeed—I humorously use the comment, because age doesn't have anything to do with it.

Statin drugs are not just cholesterol lowering drugs, statin drugs manipulate the function of your liver's ability to make cholesterol. Cholesterol is needed to make numerous cells including steroid hormones that help your organs regulate functions like blood pressure, reproductive characteristics, metabolism, immune system, and blood sugar.

The use of statins has gone up, and the percentage of Americans with high cholesterol has gone down according to the American Heart Association. So why do we see rising heart disease and not lower? Cardiovascular disease is the number one cause of death in the United States for both men and women. Yet statins are the number one class of drug prescribed. How does that even make sense? It doesn't. Notice hormone concerns, depression, and blood pressure are also going up.

If you are taking a statin drug, you may have lower cholesterol, but achieving hormonal balance will be very difficult. This is just one part of the body, but as we know, the Swiss Watch Principle means every part plays a role that can impact all the other parts. Disrupting one gear has a tremendous impact on the entire body.

CHAPTER 17

THE LIVER IS A MACHINE.

Do you remember that movie, The Horse Whisperer? The one where the guy could figure out what was going on without them being able to say it? Well, one day, I had two different follow-up appointments with two different women. They each said to me, "You are like my own Hormone Whisperer." After that I started to see it posted in comments online. I didn't ask to be called that. It's not that I don't like the nickname. It's kind of cool, but I worry people miss the point. You have made it far enough into the book to know that I don't limit myself to just looking at hormones. I disagree with the whole idea of looking at just the symptoms and treating those. I look at the whole body to find out what is happening with everything, including the hormones.

It's a Swiss watch. There are many organs that impact every piece of our overall health. What's the secret that made me The Hormone Whisperer?

The liver performs over 500 vital functions for the body.

The liver. This chapter may seem out of place, but when you understand the Swiss watch, you'll realize how crucial your liver is to everything you've just read about. But what have you been taught about the liver? Likely that it helps you detox, and alcohol can damage it. Keep reading, there is so much more to this gear in your system! You'll be looking to take care of your liver in new ways in no time!

The liver is a machine and is very important for the bigger picture. The liver performs over 500 vital functions for the body. The liver does way more than what people give it credit for. Most people just think of it as a detoxing organ, which is true. It clears out harmful toxins, like alcohol and medications, from the blood. Every day our bodies are bombarded with all kinds of toxins in our food, clothing, body products, environment, and workplace that can overload our liver. It works hard for detoxing, but it does so much more! It produces blood clotting factors and is needed for cholesterol production.

The liver stores energy, vitamins, enzymes, and minerals like iron. Did you know the liver is important for hormone conversion? It's a converting machine!

There is all this crazy stuff that happens in the liver to make up all those hormones that make up so much of who we are. They don't just show up for work, they are created by your amazing body. So, we know that cholesterol is essential for steroid hormone production. We also know cholesterol is made in the liver, which is one part of why the liver is important for healthy hormones, but it doesn't end there. After being produced in the liver, the cholesterol is excreted into the blood. That cholesterol goes off to the adrenal glands and is made into pregnenolone. Pregnenolone is known as the mother hormone. Why is it the mother hormone? Let's bring back that chart from the cholesterol chapter.

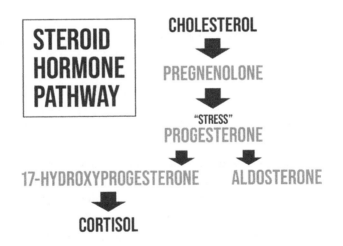

See pregnenolone is the next step on that chart, and pregnenolone has the opportunity to become all these different hormones. It is the precursor to estrogens, testosterone, progesterone, cortisol, and all the other steroid hormones. How does that happen? Once pregnenolone is produced, it goes into the bloodstream. Some of it goes to the nervous system where it is used to make myelin sheath. The main job of the myelin sheath is to protect the important stuff like your brain. If we lower cholesterol, we lower your pregnenolone which could leave your brain unprotected. The rest of your pregnenolone eventually makes its way to the testicles or adrenals where it is converted into testosterone, and to the liver where it is converted into other steroid hormones. What is happening in the body and the liver can have an impact on what those hormones become.

If we lower cholesterol, we lower your pregnenolone, which could leave your brain unprotected.

Here's a real-life example for guys that will clarify the importance of what's happening in the liver. If you have lots of testosterone production from your testicles and your adrenals, that doesn't necessarily mean your testosterone levels will be great. That testosterone eventually makes its way to the liver. The function and nutrients there can impact how it is converted there. If you have an enzyme called 5 alpha-reductase enzyme you will convert that testosterone to DHT too quickly. Too much DHT has been linked to baldness, acne, and other problems. That's not all that can go wrong once testosterone makes its way to the liver. The number one thing that accelerates the conversion of testosterone to estrogens is an enzyme called aromatase which is increased by adipose tissue. If guys produce too much of that enzyme, they will convert that testosterone they have been working hard for into estrogens and they will end up with a chest like a woman's. Sad but true, guys! Yes, you want to be sure your liver is functioning optimally.

That's why taking testosterone supplements doesn't address the actual problem. Your problem wasn't that you were short on testosterone, it's that something else is happening and that is affecting your testosterone levels. Taking a synthetic hormone doesn't get you back to normal. It might feel amazing at first, but it doesn't get you back to normal. When you have low pregnenolone, it's very common to have the other hormones low too. That's why you wouldn't want to synthetically lower your cholesterol. Like we have talked about, if you have excess cholesterol there is a stress in the body that has led to that increase in cholesterol. If a doctor synthetically lowers your cholesterol, your body can't make pregnenolone. When I see high cholesterol, I look for the cause as we know that can often be mental stress. Here's that chart that looks at hormone conversion.

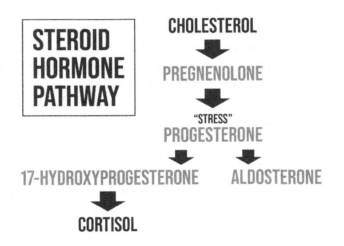

Look at that middle row where pregnenolone can either take the pathway to convert into your estrogens or it can convert into cortisol. Remember, cortisol is your stress hormone. This kicks in when you need it. Say your house is on fire. Your cholesterol should skyrocket to make pregnenolone so that your body can go into fight or flight mode. It's supposed to for you to be able to survive. Your cortisol and adrenaline are going to push to get you out of that house. That pregnenolone is going down the pathway to make those stress hormones. It's how your body was designed to survive these acute, emergency situations.

Who has the most mental stress? Ladies! Chronic mental stress leaves us in that fight or flight mode chronically. The body doesn't know the difference between whether it is a fire causing that stress or if it's because of all the everyday stresses life throws at you. It just knows stress. So, a lot of mental stress will cause the pregnenolone to be stolen for the production of your stress hormones.

This pathway is why a man can give up soda and lose twenty pounds in a week and a woman can give up soda and nothing happens. Sugar is a major stressor for men, but it's not her major stressor. That's why sometimes it doesn't matter if a woman eats good or eats poorly, she can still gain weight. Your adrenals can steal pregnenolone and stress can affect your hormones.

We can't talk about each hormone and every enzyme that affects every hormone pathway. A lot happens in the liver. What is important to know is that a lot can be happening in the liver that can show us why those hormone levels are off. Let's look at estrogen dominance specifically related to progesterone.

A lot can be happening in the liver that can show why those hormone levels are off.

What causes estrogen dominance? It could be phytoestrogens like soy, plastics, toxicity, a liver pathway issue where liver doesn't break them down, and it could be too much sugar. These all are affecting conversion change but what are they ultimately affecting? They are affecting the liver. They are affecting the liver's ability to process and regulate and normalize what the levels should be at in an optimal scenario. Our lifestyle and the 3Ts ultimately affect the liver which reflects in the hormones.

If you want to have great hormones, it's essential to have great organ function. I can't give you a magic herb that will fix your hormones. Your medical doctor can give you a drug that will force your hormones to change, but that's not a true magical fix either. A lot of hormone issues are revealed in the function of the liver. The thing is, your liver isn't kept in a bubble. Yes, if you have a bad liver, you can have bad hormones, but there is more to it than that. The gallbladder is essential for liver function. It stores the bile that breaks down the toxins from the liver. If you have a bad gallbladder, or no gallbladder, your hormones can be affected. Good stomach acid is needed to help proper gallbladder release of bile to flush out the toxins so that the liver can function properly. If you have low stomach acid, you can have affected hormones. The Swiss Watch Principle in action once again!

CHRISTY'S THOUGHTS

I remember when I learned this idea. I was sitting in one of our seminars and learning when in doubt, look to the liver. It almost always seemed like whenever you couldn't figure something out, it came back to that one organ! Now, is it always the liver? No, but the liver plays such a dynamic role in the whole body and each system of the body. Remember the Swiss watch. If I could give you any advice as a woman, I'd say lower your stress levels, but also take care of your liver. That one organ is working so hard to convert your hormones, detox your body, and communicate with other systems. Do everything you can to take care of it! Look to your toxic load from personal and home care products to the food you are eating. There are so many little things you can do to help make a big impact!

One big rule in our house is that everyone eats sauerkraut and liver every day. We are creative with how we add it to recipes, but we are also mindful in taking our glandulars and other supportive supplements to help nourish our bodies. We are doing all we can now to set our girls up with healthy habits so that they can continue on that path once they are grown.

How did I become "The Hormone Whisperer"? I didn't worry about hormones. I worried about all the things that affect your hormones. As you can see by just looking at a small part of what the liver does, it plays a major role in the hormones and the body's function overall. Just like the rest of your organ systems that make up your unique Swiss watch.

We need to look past the symptoms and to what is causing them.

We need to look past the symptoms and to what is causing them. It's sad that most readers won't find out all of this until they are already sick. Anything you do to reduce irritation or inflammation will put a lesser demand on the hormonal system.

CHAPTER 18

DETOXING IN A TOXIC WORLD.

We live in a toxic world. Some people say our bodies can handle the toxicity and don't need to worry. I disagree. The number of hazardous toxins we're exposed to daily since the Industrial Revolution has skyrocketed. About a billion pounds of pesticides are sprayed on crops every year in the U.S. We just talked about how the liver has hundreds of jobs, and one of those roles is a part of the detox process. Since the body is like a Swiss watch, those toxins aren't just impacting the liver; they are affecting the whole body. Your body can't function properly if there are a lot of toxins flowing through your body. Juice cleanses are popular, but they aren't an actual detox. If you haven't done a proper detox, overseen by a professional who understands those pathways and mechanisms, then you probably have a high toxic load.

Every choice we make is either adding to our toxic load or supporting our body. The majority of my patients aren't functioning anywhere near 100% and a lot of that starts with their toxic load. How did toxins get in your body? We are exposed to toxins daily and can acquire them from our environment by breathing, ingesting, or coming into physical contact with them. Also, most drugs, food additives, and allergens can create toxic elements in the body.

When a new patient comes into my office, they have already encountered numerous toxins adding to their very heavy toxic load. So, when I tell them they have to give up that big gulp soda they had on their way to my office, it might be painful for them, but it is just the tip of their toxic iceberg.

Let's walk through a day in the life of the average person. When their eyes flutter open in the morning, their nose is breathing toxins from the laundry soap and dryer sheet residue on their pillowcase. They stumble to the bathroom to brush their teeth with toothpaste that has fluoride, which is a known neurotoxin. Then they hop in the shower. Their shower curtain is likely made with phthalates that they will breathe in. They squirt some chemical-laden body wash in their hands and slather it on. Then they lather up their hair with shampoos that can have one of over 10,000 chemicals that are commonly used in personal care products. How many more products will they use before they leave the bathroom? That varies, but the average woman uses twelve per day, which means she's potentially been exposed to hundreds of toxins before she leaves the bathroom in the morning.

Then it is time for breakfast. The average American diet does not include a breakfast of whole, organic foods. It's usually a prepackaged meal and processed cereals. Nobody tells people the impact the ingredients in processed foods have on them. If you are eating three times a day, there are three more times you're opening yourself to toxins. Snacks? Coffee? If you aren't eating organic, whole foods then you are eating a lot of pesticides and chemicals. What kinds of pesticides and chemicals?

Did you know DDT is still used in Asia, South America, and Africa—sure, we don't use it in the U.S., but do we get food from other places? We sure do!

With the surge of GMOs that are resistant to pesticides, your breakfast likely comes with an extra serving of toxins.

Atrazine #2 pesticide is used in America with 70 million pounds used on U.S. crops each year.

Artificial colors and flavors are common in our foods. When the public becomes informed of specifics that may be harmful, they just change the name to make it more difficult to find.

MSG is not just in Chinese food. It's in lots of processed foods and is an excitotoxin (a toxin that causes an excitatory response) that has been linked to brain diseases like Alzheimer's, Lou Gehrig's disease, Parkinson's disease and learning disabilities.

Red dye #40 has been linked to hyperactivity in children. Blue dye #2 has been linked to brain tumors.

Next in my patients' day: how many pollutants did they breathe in on the drive to my office? Too many. I know, I hear it coming… "But Doc, didn't you say the body was built to detox naturally?" I did and that's still true. Here's the thing, our bodies can only handle so much before it becomes difficult for the body to naturally detoxify. Everybody has a bucket, and once your bucket is full, it gets harder to detoxify. What's your bucket? Let me explain.

There's a theory that explains this need for detoxification called "The Bucket Theory." Picture for a moment that every person has a "toxin bucket" that they are born with. At birth, some people have buckets that are somewhat empty, some are about half full, and others are nearly full. Why are some people's toxin buckets nearly full at birth? Heavy metals and other toxins can pass through the placenta to the baby. Recent studies have shown an American baby is born with approximately 280 toxins in the umbilical cord blood. That is a hard place to start from.

When a baby is born the umbilical cord will contain an average of 280 toxins.

Metal fillings, metals from vaccines and prescription drugs, cadmium from smoking or just being around cigarette smoke, lead paint, and aluminum from soda are all examples of toxins that mom could have passed to you through her placenta. If your bucket is half or nearly full at birth, would you agree with me that it would not take many more toxins to fill it up, and cause it to start overflowing? This is why we are seeing so many more sick children today! When the bucket "splashes over" you will see outward manifestations of toxic overload occurring in the body. Potential Signs of Toxic Overload:

Asthma and seasonal allergies
Cognitive problems
Depression

Anxiety
Fatigue
Headaches
Memory problems
Chronic pain
Autoimmune disease
Weight fluctuations
Eczema
Infertility
Cancer
Chemical sensitivity
Chronic infection
Diabetes
Fibromyalgia
Skin reactions
Food allergies
High blood pressure
Hormonal imbalances

We talked about how a person can start out their day encountering hundreds of toxins. If these aren't detoxed, they build up in the body. These built-up toxins can lead to many different health conditions. Even if you were born with a nearly empty bucket, with all the toxins surrounding us, it's only a matter of time before your bucket will fill up. Don't wait until your bucket overflows!

CHRISTY'S THOUGHTS

When I got pregnant, I was still in the process of changing my diet, household and body care products, and environment around me. What I didn't realize at that time was how toxic I was from my past exposure to lead paint/pipes, aluminum, and other heavy metals, as well as having a messed up immune system due to past antibiotics, and a diet that included foods that were either toxic (full of chemicals and pesticides) or toxic to me due to food allergies I didn't know I had. So, I passed toxins and an unhealthy immune system to my child. Did I have mommy guilt? Perhaps, but let me explain something that might help other mothers experiencing a similar circumstance. The fact that you are reading this book right now means that you realize that changes need to happen.

At the time that our oldest was born, we were already on a path towards homeostasis, and I knew that I was given a gift: a child. Despite all of my past health challenges. And with that gift, I was given a responsibility to continue to learn and grow in order to make sure our children would grow up healthier than me. When each of our children were born, I knew they had some toxins in their buckets. As a result, we purposefully chose to limit their toxin exposures in all areas of our lives and build their immune systems naturally. Don't look back with guilt once you learn the truth. Instead, be grateful you are learning it now and make changes moving forward. Raise your children with that 'toxin bucket' image in mind and teach them how to reduce their exposure to toxins as they are growing up so that when they are ready to have children, they won't be passing on a half or nearly full bucket of toxins to your grandchildren. If this is the first time you've heard anything about toxicity, I pray that you take this new knowledge to heart and share it with your loved ones to create a healthier future for generations to come.

Built-up hormones from a stressed-out liver can be stressors on the body.

If you take the time to assist your body in detoxification, you will help in emptying out your bucket, which will reduce the toxic stress on your body and allow it to function better. Once function is restored, your body will again be able to naturally detox itself, to some extent, on a regular basis. Now that doesn't mean after a detox that you can go back to eating non-organic, heavily processed foods or other toxic bad habits.

When you make a commitment to your health, it's a lifelong commitment. Every day your body is working to get rid of both external toxins and internal toxins. Yes, internal! Did that surprise you? Toxins can come from within. Built-up hormones from a stressed out liver can be stressors on the body. Our overall health is a reflection of the health of our cells and their ability to work together in harmony to maintain balance.

Our cells constantly take in nutrients and oxygen from the blood to work, grow, or create products, and that process produces waste. In addition to the wastes that normal function produces, we are further burdened by toxins absorbed from the intestinal tract. Poor food choices, poor digestion, and dysbiosis (parasitic, bacterial, and fungal infections) can make a mess of the intestine which makes it harder to detox. Together these absorbed toxins and the wastes produced by cells are discharged from the bloodstream into the surrounding tissues, "the cellular garbage dump," where they sit until they are transported to the organs of elimination for final disposal. Remember the cancer chapter? That's a pretty important function to keep well maintained!

You see why minimizing your toxic exposure and making sure your body is detoxing properly is so important. It's not a given, and it could very well be the reason you are sick. Or maybe you don't think you are sick. It's just old age, right? I can't tell you how many times I have had patients go through the detox, and not only did the symptoms for health problem they came in for alleviate, but they tell me they feel years younger. Sometimes twenty, thirty or even forty years younger! That's another happy side effect of being healthy.

They often lose weight too. Toxins can cause weight gain. Toxins get into fatty tissue. The body holds those toxins encased in fat as a defense mechanism, so they aren't released into the bloodstream. Once you get the toxins out of your body won't

Toxins can cause weight gain.

hold on to that fat anymore. That's long-term health benefits, not just water weight loss!

231

These are benefits you can't get from a cleanse. You wouldn't believe how many times I hear from people who have done a cleanse. You might lose some bloating, and may even get back a bit of energy, but you can't get a good detox from a cleanse. You may be surprised to hear you could actually end up making yourself even more toxic and sicker. There is a lot of confusion out there with all the fad cleanses. Let's take a look the difference between a cleanse and a detox. I have another analogy to help you to better understand!

Picture a long hallway lined with doors… now picture a janitor sweeping and scrubbing that hallway. This is what a cleanse does– it simply cleans the hallway. Now picture that same hallway lined with doors. This time the janitor not only sweeps and scrubs the hallway, but he also opens the doors and sweeps and scrubs the rooms that line the hallway. This is what a detox does. A cleanse may not require doctor supervision, but they may inadvertently harm delicate systems and leave toxins behind. The GI tract is a delicate ecosystem comprised of many kinds of bacteria. When people innocently use a cleanse to clean out their colon for example, they don't realize that they may be clearing out some good bacteria, altering the delicate ecosystem and ultimately making themselves even more sick. And the janitor didn't even do a good job cleaning!

When doing a detox with a Wellness Way doctor, we are focusing on all the detox pathways and all the organs. We are going to help clean up the whole body the best we can. You can't clean just one room or hallway and expect the whole system to function better. Eventually the mess from the other rooms spills out into the room you cleaned. Keep thinking of the Swiss Watch Principle! The body works as a whole.

Why do you need a professional to oversee your detox? While it is good to minimize your exposure to toxins by upgrading your diet to organic, whole foods and using cleaner personal care products, you can't just dive into a detox. You have a lifetime of filling and probably overflowing that bucket; there may be some damage that needs to be addressed before you go pushing toxins around.

A proficient doctor will assess and test your body to find out if it is ready for a detox. You need to know if your body is functioning well enough to handle the detox and has the nutrients to properly do so. We check for food allergies that lead to inflammation and leaky gut. The most common area we have to improve is the GI. If you are like most people, you may have gut issues. Many people have bloating, gas, diarrhea, constipation, and other signs of gut issues. What's an easy way to know if you have gut issues? Take a look at your poop. Are you pooping at least two or three times a day? Does it look like chocolate soft serve ice cream? If it doesn't, you want to get those bowels moving before stimulating your body to release toxins.

Doing that detox before your gut is ready will make for a bad day. During those first days you're drawing toxins that may be stuck in the fat tissues or other organs when you force a detox. If you try to pull those out too soon, without your GI being properly healed, all that stuff can actually leak back in the system and make you really sick.

CHRISTY'S THOUGHTS

Not so funny story about a friend who insisted that she wanted to do a detox, but to save money, she decided to go to a local health food store and buy a cheap one instead of doing the one through our office where she would be monitored by one of our doctors. She ended up in the emergency room in intense pain and became very sick as a result. The cheap 'detox' wiped out all her beneficial bacteria and caused infections that didn't exist prior to the unsupervised 'detox'. She may have saved some cash up front, but was it worth it?

I also know someone who constantly does cleanses. At one point her health had deteriorated so bad that she also ended up in the emergency room. She continued to insist that the cleanses were helping. I disagree. Moral of the stories? Your body is an intricate ecosystem of bacteria, organs and systems that work together to create homeostasis.

If something messes with the complex ecosystem, the body will try to bring itself back to homeostasis. If you are feeling 'off', don't try to guess at what will fix what's going on in your body. You need to be properly tested so you don't inadvertently make it worse.

It's not just as simple as drinking some juice and flushing the toxins out. There's important work happening there.

It may be helpful to think of the gut as a very important part of your body's detox assembly line. It's not just as simple as drinking some juice and flushing the toxins out. There's important work happening there. It's a multi-system job with three phases. A detox covers the whole body. All your organs, your blood circulation, and your lymphatic system take the detox to every corner of your body. There are some key players to support:

Liver – the main filter or cleaner
Lungs – processing O2 and H2O
Gallbladder – creates bile
Kidneys – needed for blood filtration
Intestines – microbiome has to be functioning to push the toxins out
Blood vessels and lymphatic tissue – carries out waste

All of these have to be functioning for a detox to be effective. What happens during a detox? Here are the basics:

Phase one is what we call the biotransformation phase. It's the phase where the body breaks things down from fat soluble toxins. Here's another analogy for you. You just made some really tasty bacon for breakfast. Sizzled to perfection. Instead of cleaning the pan right away, you sat down and ate that bacon. I mean if you don't eat it right away, someone else will! When you go back to clean the pan, it's crusty grease. You can't just spray water on it. You need dish soap to break it down. That's what your body does in this phase. It breaks down those fat-soluble toxins. That's why phase two is important.

Phase two is what we call the conjugation phase. This is the building things up phase. After phase one, your body is left with a bunch of broken-down metabolites that can be more toxic than the original fat-soluble toxins you started with. There are a bunch of metabolic pathways that make sure those broken-down toxins bind to natural enzymes or substances created by your liver. Some bodies are better at that than others. If your liver has been stressed for years, it can take a toll on this process. Your liver and body need support during this process to make sure those metabolites from phase one are bound so they make it to the exit. If they aren't, then they are recirculated into the body. That will make you feel very crappy.

Getting shown the door, or the excretion process, is the last important step in this process. You see this step happen every day in the way of stool, urine, and sweat. Smaller toxins that travel in the blood go to the kidneys to be filtered. Larger molecules are excreted through bile that comes from the gallbladder into the small intestine. If we are pushing toxins into the intestines, we need something to push them through the back door.

> **When you put the hard work into making sure your body is functioning, you think more about what you are exposing it to.**

Vegetables, beans, and lots of other fibrous foods are really important during the detox. We don't tell you to eat veggies because we want you to be miserable. I don't get excited about veggies, but our body needs them. I can't say this enough, if you don't get the toxins out, they can make you sick.

Can you see how critical each part of the detox process is and why it is important to support the body through each step? I bet you also see why minimizing your exposure to toxins is so important. When you put the hard work into making sure your body is functioning, you think more about what you are exposing it to.

CHAPTER 19

THE CARPENTER APPROACH TO HEALTH RESTORATION.

In our offices, we know we are often people's last hope. People have done everything else, tried everything else, and just refuse to give up. Why? They know, innately, there is a better way. There is. And honestly, I think it will shock you how simple it really is.

We talked earlier about the craziness of more illnesses now than ever before. How, for all the state-of-the-art technology and advances, we can't seem to help people recover from illnesses and get back to a healthy, vibrant life. How medicine is dictated by the insurance industry, and how sickcare and symptom management is leading people to chronic illness. Since most conditions aren't raging fires from the onset, they don't focus on eliminating the potential fire as much as managing the symptoms or just waiting until things are "bad enough" for a drug or procedure. One thing we need to better understand is that simply surviving a condition isn't restoring health.

I'm all for technology and advancements, but do you know what I'm even more in favor of? Things that work. What if we looked at a simpler way? Many of the answers we are seeking are as old as time and hiding in plain sight. But everyone is so distracted by their busy lives and the newest, shiniest answer, they miss what may have been obvious to generations past, and it was right in front of them!

Know what else is a desired side effect of restoring health? Healthy weight, skin, hair, nails... many of the things people think they are looking for.

Every day, our clinics see patients from all over the world. Because of the laws and regulations put on a D.C. and his license (remember Chapter 1?), we don't diagnose, treat, or prevent any disease. Instead, we look for the stresses to health and help restore function. That simple concept guides everything we do, including what most people have been told will never happen. We've seen autoimmune issues fade, cancer cells unexplainably shrink or go away, and healthy, vibrant lives restored. People think we are miracle workers. Nope. But the body is! Support the body to do what it was designed to do, and health is an amazing side effect!

Know what else is a desired side effect of restoring health? Healthy weight, skin, hair, nails... many of the things people think they are looking for. The answer is simple. Restore health, and the rest will come. How do you do that? I'm glad you asked.

YOU ARE WHAT YOU EAT!

I believe a significant number of the answers are here for us. It's when we let our emotions for food get in the way that it disrupts everything. I prefer my patients not to need any supplements in their cupboards, and to get all their support and nutrition from whole, organic foods. The thing is, most people have been raised to go for what is convenient, fast, and seems to taste good. Additionally, many people say it's expensive to eat healthy. Is it? I don't think so. Think about this for a minute. Many people want to trade their Oreo for an organic, gluten-free option. Of course that will cost you more! But what if you actually shopped for just good, wholesome, nutritious foods? Hint: That's typically the perimeter of the store...most of the aisles are processed foods! I'm not suggesting you swap the Oreo for an organic cookie. I'm suggesting you don't even buy it and add some good protein snack, like a bone broth smoothie or a chunk of liverwurst. Or what about some good hummus and prepared veggies? Goat cheese? See, there are options! Ahhh,

> **Many people want to trade their Oreo for an organic, gluten free option. Of course that is going to cost you more!**

but many people have an emotional attachment to those little chemically processed, nutritient deficient morsels. Trust me, I can still imagine the tastes of my childhood if I try; I just know better than to eat them!

Okay, once you decide to actually eat real, whole foods, you still have a million different opinions on what, how much, and when you should eat. Let's start with some of the "whats."

If you are to look at your body composition, it gives us a clue. Think about it this way. Your body needs building blocks to replenish and restore itself. Here's an idea that goes along with the carpenter analogy: If your house has a hole in the wall, what are you going to patch it with? Carpet? Bricks? Granite countertop? No! You'd use drywall and plaster and match your paint color. What if you had a tear in your carpet, are you filling it with plaster? Nope! You'd find the match for your carpet so that a seamless repair can be made. You need like to restore like. Make sense? If so, this next section will make sense too. But first, it's important to know what your body is composed of so that you know building blocks, or materials you need, to restore health and optimal function.

Here is an image I've used in several of my trainings, including my weekly show, *A Different Perspective*. These are rough estimates of the composition of the human body.

COMPOSITION OF THE HUMAN BODY

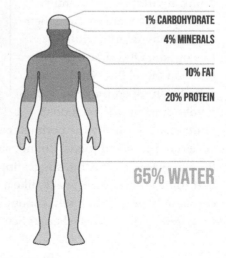

1% CARBOHYDRATE

4% MINERALS

10% FAT

20% PROTEIN

65% WATER

So tell me this, after looking at that graph: Does a high-carb, no-fat diet make sense? No!! What does your body need? Plenty of hydrating fluids, high-quality protein, fat, minerals, and carbs. For the record, the food pyramid and the recommended daily allowances (RDAs) are not even close to giving you good guidance on a healthy diet. In fact, if you eat like the food pyramid, you'll soon look like a pyramid!

> **If you eat like the food pyramid, you'll soon look like a pyramid!**

Story time! Our team loves Hawaii. I love Hawaii. Last year, I had been doing a ton of research on weight loss, muscle mass, and metabolism. I decided to ask some of the ladies who I knew were working on getting ready for their swimsuits and some time on the beach. I asked them, based on their activity levels and size, to eat between 100 and 120 grams of protein a day. These ladies were eating salmon for breakfast, bacon for lunch, burgers, steak, chicken, and my favorite, liver. Seriously, some days, they felt like they couldn't eat another bite just getting that protein in!

One day I saw one of them eating vegetables early in the day and I asked her if she'd had her protein for breakfast. Sheepishly, she admitted not enough, but realized she hadn't been eating many veggies. I told her that if she had to choose between the plant, or the thing that eats plants, I'd prefer her to eat the plant-eater! She got a good laugh and was relieved, until I told her it wasn't a free pass on no plants. We need to be sure we're getting good fiber, too! But more on that later.

What happened with all this protein? These ladies were satiated faster, performing better in the gym based on their personal workout timing (more on that coming, too!), filling out in all the ways a lady hopes to for her swimsuit while slimming down in others. What was happening? Their breast tissues were getting the building blocks to fill out, their lean muscle was burning calories 24/7, and they were seeing the results of providing the body with what it needed. Ladies are supposed to have curves, not rolls, and these ladies were noticing their hourglass figures returning.

The best part was that most of them were taking in fewer calories. The ladies' Total Daily Energy Expenditure (TDEE) was increasing by raising their physical activity and developing more muscle mass, compared to their calorie intake, so they were seeing even better results. This is a ratio (TDEE and calories in) you really have to pay attention to if you want to lose weight. Your body is going to use a certain number of calories based on your basal metabolic rate (BMR- the energy it takes to simply sustain life), thermogenesis from structured exercise programs, and thermic effect of food, known as TEF (calories needed to breakdown a specific food). Add to that the fact that you burn calories by walking, standing, taking the stairs, household chores or gardening, and leisure activities. These activities contribute to what is called your NEAT score. Non-exercise activity thermogenesis (NEAT) refers to the calories you expend in daily activities that are not structured exercise. This combination of factors is referred to as your Total Daily Energy Expenditure. They all add up! Here is a chart our team created to help you visualize what this might look like:

TOTAL DAILY ENERGY EXPENDITURE (TDEE)

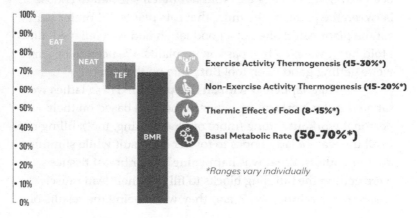

Exercise Activity Thermogenesis (15-30%*)

Non-Exercise Activity Thermogenesis (15-20%*)

Thermic Effect of Food (8-15%*)

Basal Metabolic Rate (50-70%*)

Ranges vary individually

Calories in and calories out need to be accounted for. Consider your daily activity level that contributes to your NEAT score, BMR, and workout, and if you burn more calories than you are consuming, what happens? Weight loss. It's that simple! Just be sure you are still supplying your body with all it needs to repair.

Calorie source matters because not all calories are created equal in how your body uses them! Remember that Oreo and a nutritious bone broth smoothie? The source matters in quantity, and in quality. One hundred calories of each is still 100 calories, but the effect they have on your body can vary significantly! The key is to get sufficient nutrients with fewer calories. Besides, who could eat just one Oreo? Want to know why a sufficient protein diet was a good choice for many of these ladies? They were burning calories just by digesting protein! Thermogenesis of food is another consideration. Your body easily and efficiently burns glucose. If it has to work a bit harder, it expels more calories. Protein takes more energy for your body to break down, so by choosing an energy source your body has to work for, you are holding that available glucose level lower and keeping it running.

> **Calorie source matters because not all calories are created equal in how your body uses them!**

You know what else these ladies noticed? Many of them commented on better hair, skin, and nails. These ladies were looking younger and younger! Were they all 20-year-olds to begin with? Nope! Many of these ladies were well into their 30s and 40s. They'd been pregnant, nursed babies, and "tried everything else before!" Beauty secret? Maybe…unless you know what your body needs!

Speaking of what your body needs, and hair, skin, and nails… one thing that has made a huge spike in popularity lately is collagen. Is collagen good for you? It has benefits. Does your body need it? It needs some of the amino acids to help recovery and repair. Some of these ladies, when they were getting tired of bacon and steak (can you believe it?), tried to get their fill on bone broth and collagen. We love that around the office, and in fact we have our own brand. I told many of them that they had to stop relying on that as an easy out, because we still needed more of a specific amino acid that comes in higher concentrations in other protein sources. They could have it, sure, but that wasn't going to make up the most of their protein. Why? A little essential amino acid called leucine.

Back to the building blocks! Amino acids are the literal building blocks available in protein. Your body breaks proteins down into these amino acids to take and rebuild as needed. There are twenty-one amino acids that are required by the human body: Nine of them are essential. Essential amino acids are the ones you need to take in through your diet. Your body can't synthesize them from other nutrients. Leucine is an essential amino acid for muscle protein synthesis. Your body needs leucine to create muscle.

I encouraged these ladies to be taking in good, high-quality, bioavailable leucine sources. I can hear it now, "But Doc, I don't want to look like a body builder!" Ahhh, let me tell you why lean muscle is so important.

Each year, one in four elderly Americans report falling each year. In fact, falls are the cause of the most fatal and non-fatal injuries each year. According to the CDC, nearly 4,000 adults die each year due to the injuries sustained by falls. This doesn't account for those who don't recover well from a traumatic fall; we know that number is much higher. Now, let's look at an elderly person's diet. High in protein? Unlikely. So, according to what we've already discussed, we can see that their skeletal muscles (the ones that help us balance and hold us upright) are weakened. What do you think happens to an elderly person who is unable to adequately and safely support and balance themselves? They fall. So, while I may have been helping these ladies get ready for their swimsuits and beach time, I was really helping them to look ahead 30, 40, 50 years, or more, to create the body they'll want to live in as a healthy elderly person! Protein is important for longevity.

Ladies aren't the only ones who need more protein. Guys need to be hitting protein hard too! I like to recommend that people take in about one oz of protein for every pound they weigh. Now, considering their BMR and NEAT scores is important too. If you are looking for weight gain, loss, or management, you need to be focused on that balance of calories in and calories out. Don't forget the leucine! I generally recommend about 2.5 grams per meal or higher to make sure you're getting enough.

When consuming meats, make sure you are getting organic, grass-fed, pasture-raised (mammal-source), free-range (poultry and eggs), and wild-caught (fish). Remember, organ meats, especially liver and liverwurst, are your highest and most nutrient-dense sources. Everyone who comes to my house has a serving: It's a Flynn house rule!

WHAT ABOUT PLANT-BASED PROTEINS?

Can you be a healthy vegetarian or vegan? You can. But you are going to have to put a whole lot more effort into your food than meat eaters will. Why? The protein in plants, even those high-protein sources, are so bound within the fibers of the plant that you would have to consume so many more calories and work to diligently prepare them so they are bioavailable to digest. To absorb 120 grams of protein, you'd likely have to take in nearly a minimum of 200 grams from certain plant sources. It really is harder.

So how do you calculate protein intake accurately, especially on a plant-based diet? The digestible indispensable amino acid score (DIAAS) is a calculation based on the total amino acid content in a protein along with digestibility and absorbability. Think of it this way. There may be a lot of protein in a specific food, but how much of that is actually available to use?

Keep in mind when using plant proteins that the label will show you how many grams of protein are in the plant itself. Now, you have to take into account that binding to the fiber, and how well you are digesting and absorbing it. You can't just read a label and assume that's how much protein you'll be taking in. And don't forget those amino acids!

For those who are looking to use plant sources as a replacement or an addition to meat sources, I've put together a list of my favorites:

- Hemp
- Chia Seeds
- Lentils
- Chickpeas (garbanzo beans)
- Black Beans
- Pinto Beans
- Green Peas
- Brussels Sprouts
- Pistachios
- Quinoa

Many people ask me why soy isn't on this list. Well, soy has certain things I like to avoid, (levels of phytoestrogens) that may have an effect on hormone levels. Also, soy is one of the highest GMO crops. In fact, 95% of soy in the U.S. is GMO.

THE ONE THING ALL HEALTHCARE PROFESSIONALS AGREE ON

I can hear it now, "Doc said I don't have to eat any veggies!" That's not what I said. In fact, if you don't eat the right veggies, or even some fruits, or other plants, it'll be a bad day. Here is the one thing I found that no health care professional will disagree on: You need fiber. Not your grandma's bran flakes; but real, good, plant-based fiber. Let me give you a hint, though. The RDAs were not created to promote health, they're just there to keep you from massive deficiencies. The RDA for women is 25 grams of fiber, and for men, it's 38. Those are way too low! I like to see women somewhere near 40 grams and men at about 50 grams.

Why is fiber so important? First of all, let's be clear on what fiber is and what it does. Fiber is a type of carbohydrate that your body uses in digestion. Carbs are typically broken down into glucose molecules for the body to use as an energy source. When you are reading labels, you subtract the fiber from the total carbs to see what is left that will affect your available glucose levels. Generally speaking, fiber helps

You need fiber. Not your grandma's bran flakes, but real, good, plant-based fiber.

you feel fuller, better absorb nutrients, clear your GI of waste, and supports a healthy blood sugar. How?

There are two types of fiber: Soluble and insoluble. Your body needs both. Soluble fiber dissolves and creates a gel-like substance. This soluble fiber helps regulate bacteria and a good microbial balance by giving those bacteria what they need to feed off of. Soluble fiber helps food to be absorbed as it's moving through the GI tract. Other benefits from this process include supporting a healthy blood sugar (available glucose level) and cholesterol. We've talked about how important those factors are to health!

So, what is insoluble fiber? Consider this, your GI is where nutrients are absorbed, biochemical processes occur, and waste is carried out. But that waste needs some help to be carried out. That is where insoluble fiber comes in. It adds water and bulk so that the waste can be carried out of the body. If you've been around The Wellness Way, you know that GI health is crucial to overall health. Getting the gut in order is usually one of our first steps for most patients.

It's no secret that my favorite source of fiber is

sauerkraut. The benefits are huge! Good fiber, probiotics, vitamins C and K1... seriously, sauerkraut is way underappreciated. Choosing the right sources of fiber is also important. Here is a list I've put together to help my audiences and patients make the best choices for themselves:

Fruits: Avocado, blackberries, raspberries
Vegetables: Mashed sweet potatoes, artichokes, Brussels sprouts
Nuts, seeds, & legumes: Chia seeds, sunflower seeds, lentils, almonds, chickpeas
Other high fiber foods: Cacao nibs, dark chocolate, coconut flakes, psyllium husk powder

FASTING AND NON-EATING STRATEGIES

It's no secret that I have people who love what I say, and people who can't stand what I say. This one topic has certainly triggered so many people. Fasting has become such a hot trend that people ask my opinion all the time. Here it is: Clinically, I've found men should fast 1-3 days quarterly. I wouldn't encourage women to fast like that. And if they need to, it should be under the guidance and care of a doctor who is very familiar with their lab markers, especially their hormones. Why do I say this? Remember what stress does to a body?

Fasting is a physiological stressor, it creates a similar effect on the body as exercise, screaming at others, running from predators, or being anxious. It reduces blood sugar, insulin, and inflammation, but does quite the opposite for cortisol. Many people are familiar with the infamous hormone associated with stress and belly fat. Cortisol increases adrenaline and prepares the body for survival in a stressful or dangerous situation. These functions of cortisol are part of a normal, healthy stress response. But one thing, the body shouldn't be in that state constantly! Chronic stress is bad. Acute stress is a normal response because the levels of hormones are created to shift back to normal levels relatively quickly.

When people talk about fasting, often they're not using the right terms. It takes 2-3 days for certain foods to pass from mouth to rectum. To constitute a fast, you would want no food in the system. Dietary restrictions, caloric restrictions, and time-restricted eating is difficult to equate to fasting. That does not mean they aren't beneficial for some people, or don't have their place. It's just important to know what you are doing.

One thing that would be more beneficial than fasting, especially for women, is eating the proper food as fuel at the right time of day, in the right ratios for you and your needs, and make sure not to eat too many calories compared to your TDEE. Start with the right protein and fiber and then take into consideration what else you need. How does your body run best? Fats? Carbs? How many calories? Understanding your individual needs is what will support your individual health! Some people like to consider time-restricted eating. I get it, it helps you stay on track and gives the body time to "rest and digest." If this is something that helps you, I'd suggest eating during the 8am-4pm window as a start and see how that does for your needs.

What would be more beneficial than fasting, especially for women, is eating the proper food as fuel at the right time of day, in the right ratios for you and your needs.

NO SUGAR CHALLENGE

Each year we run a No Sugar Challenge in the month of January. I hear it every single time, "But Doc! Our bodies run on sugar!" Yep, you're right! Glucose is the easiest form of fuel for your body to run on. But the challenge is that most people eat way, way too much sugar, even when they limit it to fruits and natural forms. When glucose is too high for too long, it contributes to metabolic syndrome which contribute to all conditions. When you reduce your sucrose (glucose + fructose), the fancy name for "sugar," you can reduce many of those risk factors.

What happens when you limit that readily available glucose? First of all, you are likely breaking some bad eating habits. Your brain and body will want that sugar for the first several days and you may feel miserable as you work through that. Don't give up! This is a huge indicator that you were likely consuming too much sugar to begin with. Your body is learning to use alternate fuel sources, that takes training, both mentally and physically.

Secondly, your body is going to need to adapt and start breaking down extra adipose tissue (fat) and other reserves for energy. Sometimes people feel flu-like symptoms when they switch over to no sugar, and their body starts using those reserves. Know why? Your body is brilliant and protects itself by capturing toxins in adipose tissues so that it doesn't circulate. What happens when you start burning that adipose tissue? Those toxins get pushed out. As long as you are supporting those liver pathways, they can be eliminated. That's important! If that doesn't happen, it's a bad day because those toxins can start circulating again.

BECOME YOUR BEST TRAINER

Exercise is one of those strange things. It's almost like every style or form has their own little cult-like following. Tell me I'm wrong. Think about people who do these specific types of exercise and how dedicated they are to their "practice." Yogis. Cross-fitters. Dancers. Pilates enthusiasts. Runners. Martial artists. Gym rats. You know these people are convinced their form of exercise is perfect and good for everyone. Don't believe me? Ask them, they'll tell you! But I have a question for you. Is it? Is there a single workout style that is good for everyone at all times? No.

Why? The little thing we come back to in every single chapter. Hormones. The biggest thing I want you to take away is that everyone should be moving every day. Every day? Every day. The type of activity you do (I love resistance for most people) and how intensely you do it should be driven by what you know about your hormones and the inflammation response your body is experiencing. If you don't know what that is, you

> **The biggest thing I want you to take away is that everyone should be moving every day. Every day? Every day.**

could be setting yourself up for the opposite results you are hoping for and might even through off your body.

Let's start with guys. Why? Same reason as before; you're simple. Guys, go hard. Get in the gym and just crank it and build that testosterone and muscle tissue. Hard work is good for guys. You don't have to worry about tanking your hormones, in fact, working out is one of the best ways to increase testosterone! Yes, a person can over train, there is research to show that, but I think we can all agree that the overwhelming majority of men need to work out more.

Next easiest group is post-menopausal women. Why? They are mostly governed by progesterone and testosterone. They can exercise a bit more intensely than cyclical women as long as they keep their nutritional intake up especially their proteins but remember: don't over consume calories.

Okay, cyclic women, we've got some more thoughts for you. Why? Hormonal deficiencies impact you so much harder and faster. If you deplete fat tissue too far and overwork your adrenals, you'll affect your hormones. How can you tell? You start skipping your period and if you do have it, you have less uterine lining to shed and less blood flow. Remember your period should be no less than 5 days, but closer to 6 or 7 days. I know women hate to hear that, but it's really important. You don't want any of that tissue left behind. Support your system nutritionally so you have the proper building blocks and energy sources to properly fuel your workouts and hormones.

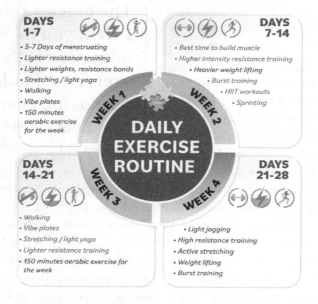

I've had ladies love this and ladies hate this. But you know what? When they tried it, they saw the difference and realized it not only helped their health, but it also reduced the mental stress of having to be a cross-fit crazy person every day, whether they felt like they were dying or not! It also helped them understand how to actually use activity to lose weight, gain lean muscle, and do it without all the stress and competition. I realized that many women feel like they are failing. Let's face it, ladies are supposed to have curves. You know what most workout crazed women look like? Pre-pubescent boys. And call me crazy, but I'm sure that's not what guys consider attractive! Ladies, let me say it again, you are supposed to have curves. If you reduce your adipose tissue (too low of body fat %) too far, you'll affect your hormones levels. Now you don't want excessive fat rolls, understandably: That's neither healthy nor attractive, but your curves are what give you that feminine shape men are attracted to.

This chart and concept is so important, the ladies in our office refer to it daily. I think most people would be shocked if they heard the daily conversations. In reality, it's a little awkward for new people when they come to work for us but haven't been a part of The Wellness Way before. The open talk about a lady's cycle has been known to drop a few jaws and cause some faces to blush. But they get over it, ladies get healthier, and guys learn a thing or two about supporting the women in their lives.

We have a gym in our headquarters. I noticed many people were working later and starting to neglect getting out and getting active. Instead of incentivizing them with reduced gym memberships, I just put in a full gym of our own! Reduce the stress and make it simple for everyone! Before work, during lunch, after work, weekends, that place is used all day, every day. The ladies walk into the gym and know what to do. Is it Stairmaster day? Weights? Cycling? Light stretching? If they have questions, they'll unapologetically walk up to one of our doctors who is also working out, or another team member (guy or gal) who is more familiar with exercise and the chart and announce which week they are on and ask for help. You know what's not in that room? Judgement because she's not pushing herself harder than she should. Ladies, if you can get over the fact that you have a cycle and that it impacts what you should be doing, you'll only set yourself up for better results! If you don't have someone to ask, you can always bet resistance training is a good, safe bet. Getting oxygen to the muscles and tissues is so important. Just monitor that heart rate based on where you ought to be.

Let's walk through why this graph is important, and how to use it.

Days 1-7: This is the part of your cycle where you are bleeding. Tell me this, do you want to go for a run? No. Why? Your body simply does not have the hormonal reserves and production to sustain more than light activities. You have such little hormone at this time--no progesterone or testosterone--and estrogens are just starting to build. It is so important to keep your heart rate and stress levels low. Even exercise is a stress on the body. Just get oxygen to the muscles and focus on supporting your body so that next week, and later in the month, you have all you need to do more intense workouts. During this week, consider simply standing on a vibe plate, a small trampoline, yoga, stretching, light walking, lower resistance training. It's good to give those muscle some stress, but do not overdue it this week.

Day 7-14: Hit it hard! This is a week you can handle stress. You'll feel like you can take on the world and keep going. This is the easiest time build muscle because testosterone levels start to come up. Go for those high intensity workouts, higher resistance training, raise your heart rate, and sweat.

Days 14-21: Remember week one? This is your repeat of that week. This time, progesterone is supposed to counteract the estrogens that are increasing and keep that healthy balance. Progesterone is a hormone that can easily run down that pathway to cortisol and cortisone. Get back to a very similar exercise routine in week one.

Days 21-28: This is your wild-card week and depends on how well you took care of the other weeks. Remember earlier in the women's chapters? Hormones are going to drop down again so the cycle can restart. If you have week 2 energy, push a bit more like week 2 so you can help those hormones come down and restart the cycle. If you are depleted, you'll know it. You still need to help your body prepare for the beginning of your cycle, but don't push so hard that you go into a prolonged cortisol and cortisone response.

Ladies, I know this may be a change from what you've been taught. But trust me. Try it. You will have to shift your mindset, but the benefits will be worth it!

GET YOUR BEAUTY REST!

Remember earlier when I was talking about protein and all the ladies discovered they were seeing benefits beyond weight loss? Skin, hair, nails, youthfulness? Know why? Repair and restoration: They were literally giving their body what it needed to rebuild. Guess what, there is something to the old thought of beauty sleep as well! Why? It's the time of day your body is repairing, restoring, and rebuilding. Same concept. Let me give you a little insight, third shift work is now considered a known carcinogen. Your body needs the appropriate rest at the right times, which is based on your circadian rhythms. Your body knows the rhythm it needs to function. Support that, and you support life.

Think about it this way. What did our ancestors do when the sun went down? Sit in artificial light and watch flickering screens? No, they sat around a fire and allowed their body to begin the resting process, and then slept in total darkness. What did they do when the sun came up? They got up and started their day outside and in the sunlight! I encourage people to get up in the morning, get their feet on the ground, and tilt their face to the sun just to reset that proper rhythm, and let the lights go down in the evening as the sun goes down.

I run 100 miles an hour and many people wonder if I ever sleep. Of course I do, but I also know how to use my circadian rhythm to its advantages and support it so that it can support me. This concept can help you get more out of your day...even if you spend more of it sleeping!

Men, you need roughly around 8 hours of sleep per night. If a guy gets to bed by 9-10 and gets up about 5-6am, he should be good to go and take on the day. But you better understand this, your wife needs more sleep, and you better not shame her for it.

Ladies, I know you have a long list of things to do, but you need 8-10 hours of sleep. And not just any 8-10, but a very specific window. You use your hormonal reserves through the day and rebuild them at night. I'm sorry, but you don't have testicles that help you rebuild those depleted hormones like guys do. The best time to begin building that reserve is at about 9pm through 1-2am. Now, don't think you can get up at 1-2 am! Just know that if you go to bed later and stay in bed for a full 8-10 hours, you miss that vital time for your body to release those specific hormones. Cortisol and other hormones start to increase around 3am. If they spike too quickly, you'll wake up too early and set off your rhythm. We see this happen to many women who have trouble regulating their cortisol and their blood sugar.

When you learn to support and regulate normal blood sugar throughout the day, it will help with cortisol through the night. Hormones should peak around 6-8am signaling your body that it is time to wake up. Considering all the work the body has to go through during sleep to rest and repair, the ideal sleep time for a woman is during the window of 9pm until 6 or 7am. This regular sleep pattern should help you feel more clear minded and get you the necessary sleep to rebuild the hormone levels you need to make it through the day.

IT ALL COMES BACK TO ONE THING: STRESS

What is the one thing we keep hammering on? Stress. Exercise, living, eating, digesting, repairing, all of this puts a stress on your body. When you're able to manage these stressors, you will be better prepared for the ones you may not be able to control.

Ladies, you need to get stress under control. Physically, mentally, and emotionally. You need to give yourself a chance to repair so that your body can handle the natural stressors of daily life. Guys, you need to help her out. Your body is designed to handle it better.

Remember, health is a side-effect of lifestyle. Your health and the choices you make to support it are in your hands. Sometimes there's something else going on. That is when you need to reach out to someone, like one of our Wellness Way doctors or health restoration coaches, and get those levels properly tested to get you back on the right track.

CHAPTER 20

SAY IT...
I DISAGREE.

Imagine a wilting plant. What do you think that plant might need to perk back up? Water, or maybe sunlight. Why didn't you say drugs or surgery? Why didn't you say horse hormones? Most people understand more about how to take care of a plant than their own body. That's frustrating for me. Traditional doctors do their best to manage symptoms and minimize pain. It's honestly amazing what they can do, but what they're never taught to do is support the body to bring it back to normal function. It's not how they are trained to look at or approach a health condition. They are trained to go in with their ax and hose to do what they were taught to do, to save your life. Both sides of this conversation are important—stopping the fire and rebuilding the house. I disagree with simply putting out the fire.

Every day, couples are told they will not be able to have a baby. Then there are the patients who hear they need to be on a drug for their high cholesterol. Girls are told birth control is the answer to their period problems. People are told they are fat because of genetics. Divorce rates are increasing because society tells us men and women are the same. Menopause is a change that is feared. Men are told testosterone goes down as they age. Women are told there is nothing wrong with them even though they have a laundry list of symptoms. I disagree with all of this and so much more. What is your perspective after reading this book?

Don't you agree that there needs to be another approach? One that builds the body? I want this approach to be known all over. Everyone deserves it! You deserve individual care that treats you, not just the average person. Your body is a Swiss watch with different gears and unique makeup; that means an individual set of hormones. It means individual factors and individual circumstances. Now that you

You deserve individual care that treats you, not just the average person.

know a different way to look at the body, you have powerful information that can change the future of your health.

I have one more story of someone who dared to disagree in one of the most heartbreaking times of her life.

PATTY'S STORY

After 11 years of infertility, exploratory surgeries, and rounds of IVF, I was feeling done. It was hard wanting to be pregnant, seeing pregnant strangers, or being with a friend who was expecting a baby. I had been told by the IVF doctors I'd never be able to carry a baby in my womb. They told me I would have to look into a surrogate or adopt. I wanted to have a hysterectomy. If I couldn't use my female organs, I didn't want them.

When we had found The Wellness Way and Dr. Patrick, a cancelation enabled us to get in right away. I knew it was meant to be!

We learned a whole new lifestyle at The Wellness Way. The approach was completely different. From all that we learned, I have referred my sister, a neighbor, people with cancer, and those with other health challenges. While some people are opposed to trying anything different, others have great results with The Wellness Way.

We had several people who were skeptical and told us it wouldn't work. I faced my own challenge. I worked in the dairy industry. Due to my allergies, I had to eliminate dairy from my diet. I often heard "don't bite the hand that feeds you;" but I had to do what was right for my body.

When I share my Wellness Way story, a lot of people are concerned about insurance coverage. I tell them all it's worth it. If this is what you want, and this is your dream in life, then there really is no dollar amount. When we went through IVF, we spent tens of thousands of dollars. All the medications were out of pocket as well. When I talked to my insurance company about IVF, I was told having a child isn't a necessity of life and they wouldn't cover it. Now, I tell people to put that money toward fixing your body the right way. Let it work the way it should and treat it right. You only have one body.

Since the time of publishing, Patty had baby number three!

HOPE RESTORED

I want to share more of Patty's story with you. As she and her husband, Josh, tried to start their family, they faced some heartache. Like many married couples, Patty and her husband Josh tried to get pregnant. After trying for eleven years, guess what happened, nothing. She went to the medical doctors. They only have two tools. They gave her medications; did she get pregnant? No. She didn't. So, they only had one tool left, they decided to do IVF therapy. They extracted three eggs from her ovaries and fertilized them, then they implanted one. Any guess how much that cost? $20,000. Insurance covers nothing.

Patty and Josh paid the $20,000 and it did not work. They implanted the second egg for $20,000 and that didn't work. The doctors told Patty and her husband that they had one more egg left, and they felt bad for her since she had already spent $40,000, so they'd do the last one for $5,000. But before they did this, the doctors said they'd heard about this guy in Green Bay, Wisconsin. They were talking about me! They didn't really know what I do, but they told her, "He gets crazy results."

Patty and her husband came into The Wellness Way. As we were going through her medical records, I asked her some very basic questions. "Did they test your hormones?"
"No."

Well, they actually had tested one of them, but it was incomplete testing. We tested all her hormones and found the imbalance. I started the process of finding the triggers and what she needed to do to balance her hormones. It took time to rebuild her body. After nine months we retested her. She was regaining healthy levels of hormones; I sent her back to her doctor. They

did the last in-vitro and she got pregnant. I was so happy
for her and Josh!

Here's what followed. Medicine has standards they do
with everyone. One of the standards they do with IVF is to give
the woman hormone shots. They have to force the body to keep
the pregnancy. This is a standard because, unless the mother is
working with a doctor like those in our Wellness Way network,
the body hasn't been brought to a place of healthy function.
Standard medicine is trying to help, and make sure they
manipulate those hormone levels to maintain the pregnancy.
Josh, Patty's husband, called me, concerned about the shots.
"Doc, is this okay?" I told him, "Her labs are normal; the shots
now will make her abnormal again, and she'll get sick. "

She went back to the doctor, shared her concerns, and
the doctor told her "Dr. Patrick is hurting you, don't go back to
him. You have to do this. If you do not, we won't take care of
you." You know what? He was trying to make sure she did what
he knew, based on
his experience.

See guys, they don't see the body like we do, so they
don't understand this approach. They haven't been trained to
and some might even stop you
from asking questions. A doctor
who doesn't allow you to
question his approach is wrong.
What have those other doctors
done? They've tried, but their
thinking is focused on the
fire. We rebuild the body and

> **A doctor who doesn't allow you to question his approach is wrong.**

support the body's natural ability to heal. This leads to places
traditional medicine is unfamiliar with.

So, what happened with Patty? She was scared so she
listened to them and got the shots. Six weeks later, in October,
that baby died. My heart broke for her. The doctor conclusively
told her, "You can't have children," and left. He had nothing

left to offer her. Imagine how she felt in that moment. She had trusted this doctor, and he had no answers for her.

She went into a deep depression after she lost the baby. Josh texted me and called me often saying, "I can't get Patty out of bed she's so depressed." I told him to leave her be, she had to get her stress down. It was a normal reaction both physically and mentally to what she had just been through. She lost a baby and the idea of a family—she was going through tremendous physical stress. A month later I hadn't heard from them. Then Josh reached out to me again. "Doc, Patty's finally getting up and around. You made the most sense to us even when the other doctors didn't understand your thinking. My wife was the happiest and healthiest when she was with you. I understand we can't have a baby, but I'd rather have my wife happy and healthy than sick with no child."

I told him, "I know what the doctors said, but I disagree. Don't tell your wife that though. She doesn't need to hear that right now. We need to remove the stressors and get her body functioning." Her body was struggling with the synthetic hormones she had been injected with. We had to detox her and build her hormones back properly. That detox was painful for her; there was a lot that needed to be pulled out. She felt like she was going to die. A detox can be very hard when you are properly pulling all of the toxins. February 8th, I called Patty so we could redo her labs. She said that she and Josh were going to go on vacation to Mexico for three weeks. I told her to call me when she got back.

March came around and all of a sudden, I got a text message from Patty. She said, "Dr. Patrick, I was at work today and my boobs were sore, I was tired, and I got nauseous, so I went to Walgreens and I bought seven pregnancy tests and they are all positive. How did that happen?!" I told her she was a little old for the talk about the birds and the bees and she should know how it happened! I laugh every time I tell that part of the story!

Every once in awhile , Patty would send me a picture of her son, "Joshua wanted to say hi to his favorite doctor!" Why am I his favorite doctor? Because their story had a happy ending for them, but their story was far from easy. The other doctors had given up hope and offered his parents no hope of having children. Their thinking and philosophy were different than the one Patty and her husband needed. They may get many accolades and high recognition at their jobs, but does their thinking get you where you truly want to be? Back to normal function and health?

There is no other approach? I disagree! I'm so saddened by people being sick, infertile, unhappy, and divorced. I want to live in a world where rates of cancer, heart disease, and all common, chronic diseases are actually decreasing. We have to change the direction that we are going in and it has to start somewhere. Even if that means simply saying I disagree.

DARE TO DISAGREE

People are uncomfortable with the concept of disagreement. It has negative connotations, and even just the thought can bring on feelings of anxiety, anger, stress, and tension. However, disagreement does not have to be a bad thing – in fact, when done respectfully, it's actually a very

> **There is no other approach? I disagree.**

good thing! Why do I say that? Because the ability to disagree and walk through constructive conflict is a gift – it means you have a choice. It means we have the opportunity to learn and grow and pursue new things. Things that may be different from the norm.

At the beginning of the book, I brought up the idea that many people woke up during COVID. They saw the tyranny and control government and pharma were imposing on their lives. From their work to how they got healthcare, which stores they could shop at, who they could see for Christmas, and whether they could be in their dying parents' hospital room for final goodbyes. As horrible as that whole ordeal was, it brought an awakening to just how much some people are willing to turn over to the government and non-elected, imposed figures.

Sometimes when you stand up and dare to disagree, you'll be faced with pushback and conflict. Conflict isn't bad! We have to get over the emotion that it is. In reality, conflict allows for the discussion of disagreeing perspectives. If you choose to avoid conflict, you will likely be forced to choose to live quietly, accepting what other people think you should have or believe. How is that a life?

I have been standing up and disagreeing for years. But, during all the COVID lockdowns, my choice to stand up gained a lot more attention. I created a bubble for my employees and family. In a state gone crazy, our company had no social distancing, no masking, no vaccines...unless they were chosen. Guess how many people in that circumstance chose to follow those ridiculous, imposed mandates or even the suggestions made. None of them. We even had a Christmas gathering for the people in our community, complete with Santa, since he wasn't visiting the malls! We had hundreds of community members show up. We got media attention, all right! We were labeled as "super spreaders" and dangerous.

Just a few months later, the FBI showed up at my home. They were actually pretty kind. I almost wondered if they thought this was crazy stuff as well! They asked me a question, "Do you believe you are a danger to society?" My answer was easy. "No! I believe I am good for society!" You see, without the ability to disagree, government and large corporations become dangerous, not the populace who stand up to the tyranny! They left, but the police were at the end of my driveway for another twelve hours.

I picketed alongside nurses who had previously thought we were crazy, I supported their right to choose the vaccine! I fought legal battles for others with my own money. We won every one of them. Those legal battles protected families, children, and parents from the dangers of mandates and gave them the ability to keep their jobs and go to school. Why? I understand I have the finances to fight some of these battles that others can't. I can back it financially, I just need others to rise up and continue the fight, too!

But no matter how many times law enforcement shows up at my home or place of business, no matter how many family disagreements I get in, no matter how many legal battles, no matter how many of our media platforms get taken down (too many to keep track of!), I will continue to stand up and disagree. Why? Because if I don't, who will? I'm not willing to allow my family's future and health to be dictated by the government or corporations! And sometimes, when one stands up, many others find the courage to join in. Then, we aren't a danger to society but a force for good!

Imagine knowing what you know now after going through this book, and not having the option to disagree. Imagine being told nothing can be done, and the door is shut forever. Imagine a doctor looking at you and your very real symptoms, telling you it's all in your head, and it's the end. Imagine being handed a laundry list of prescriptions with side effects worse than the actual illness, and being told it doesn't matter, you'll be fine, and there's simply no other options. Maybe that hopeless scene has already been a part of your story – it surely has been for tens of thousands of other people and is one of the reasons I am so passionate about this topic. This, right here, right now. This is the part of the story where we get to make a change.

Health is a very emotional topic, and understandably so. It's extremely personal and can have consequences that can literally destroy lives; be it financially, emotionally, physically, or a combination of all three. People can become extremely defensive about health decisions and rely heavily on emotions. Having come this far in your understanding, however, let me ask you a question: do you think the traditional medical way of

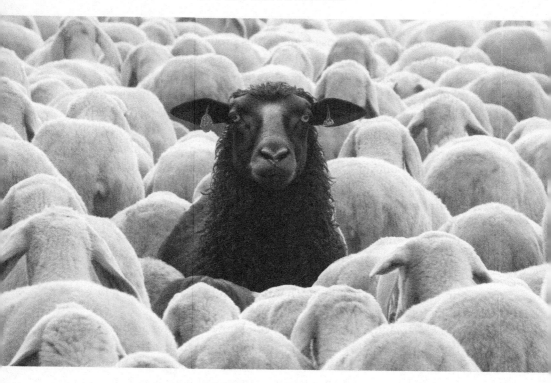

People become extremely defensive about health decisions and rely heavily on emotions.

thinking has been bringing us closer to health? Emotional as it may be, looking at the statistics, there is no question: the fire department is excellent, but we are sorely lacking in carpenters. Our emergency care is second to none, but if we are increasingly dying from long-term, chronic conditions, something is still wrong. We are not healthy.

Taking the conventional path is easy. If you don't count the frustration, heartache, and hit-and-miss results, you will find it a comforting path. You will be like the vast majority of the herd, and people are very comfortable with being a part of a crowd and going along with the masses. Everyone going one way, traveling together with little resistance along the clearly marked path. Here's the problem though – where's the herd going? Are they taking you where you really want to go? I think if we all think long and hard over the last several years, we can be more honest with ourselves and that answer.

In the picture above, there's a sheep thinking differently. He has his head raised high, and clearly has ideas that differ from the herd. While the other sheep are being blindly led, that single sheep is changing his story. This is how I picture life. So many people are blindly following a path, in the pursuit of health. The path is a series of misinformation, bad habits, and poor health advice, and however well-intended, the intent doesn't matter because the actual results are disastrous. It's a bleak picture, but that's what makes this exciting – the story isn't over.

I said it at the beginning of the book, and I'll say it again here: I am very proud of my profession and study of chiropractic. The principles and philosophies I learned are the foundation of all I have done. Anytime I look at studies, data, and research, my training gives me insights to see things differently. I've heard many times, "You aren't a real doctor, you're just a chiropractor." I chuckle, shake my head, then go and continue to guide others as they change their lives with the health restoring principles based on simply physiology and chiropractic philosophy. I'm not just a chiropractor. I am a proud chiropractor.

In the picture above, I think you know which sheep I identify with – the one thinking differently! I hope by now I have provided enough evidence and provoked enough thought that you are thinking differently too. Unlike the image though, there is more than just one who is bold. There are many of us.

This is where the story changes, for the better!

Actually, there are hundreds of thousands of us – across the country, and across the globe, all thinking differently and taking a stand. Realizing there's more to be done, realizing there are different, better answers, and getting incredible results as we go. This is where the story changes, for the better! Not just my story, your story. Your story is so important! Not just to you, but to everyone around you. Your story reaches your loved ones and community and has the power to change lives. This is where we impact not only our generation, but generations to come. Now, more than ever, it's time to take a stand, think differently, and say, "I disagree!"

DO YOU DISAGREE, TOO? NOW WHAT?

Just because the book is done doesn't mean this story is over.
Connect with us on our social channels. Visit our website for
more life changing content, find a clinic near you, or attend
an event. We are excited to keep empowering you to think
differently, and to say, "I disagree!"

DR. PATRICK FLYNN

drpatrickflynn.com

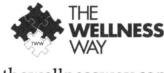

thewellnessway.com

Follow us for up to date information, articles,
videos, recipes, and events.

Made in the USA
Las Vegas, NV
10 May 2024

89733091R00148